THE EVOLVING HUMAN AND THE FUTURE WORLD

THE EVOLVING HUMAN AND THE FUTURE WORLD

By

PAVAN RAINA

MD PUBLICATIONS PVT LTD
NEW DELHI

Published by

MD Publications Pvt Ltd
B/231-E, Greater Kailash - I
New Delhi-110048.
E-mail : contact@mdppl.com
Website : www.mdppl.com

Showroom

"MD House"
11, Darya Ganj
New Delhi-110002
Tel. : +91-11-23268645, 23271378
Fax : +91-11-29235450

ISBN 81-7533-096-1

Printed by

Times Press
910, Jatwara Street, Darya Ganj
New Delhi-110002.

INDEX

PREFACE

The manuscript “Evolving Human And The Future World” is the original thought of the author and has no direct relevance to any historical study of present or past. The author thinks that any discovery or invention made by human is nothing that did not exist and was always there but humans were unable to see it. One brilliant human starts seeing that invisible to others till that moment and when he communicates scientifically or philosophically or by any other means there are others who start receiving the message and gradually with involvement of more brilliant brains the subject starts making a shape. With passage of time, the progress of the message through number of modifications becomes a well-known fact to every person.

There are scores of content on the subject of evolution and human civilisation and well documented historical facts from the ancient past to the present. In the present book the author has assumed a zero reference state of human when he was just equivalent to any other animal present in the mental make up and thus his methodology for the survival was mere on natural animal instincts. What made the first change in the brain of such human animal has not been stated as that does not interest the subject but how the brain starts seeing the things has been explained.

Some simple questions such as who am I? Why have I come in this world? What is happening in the world? What is my part? Could crop in many not because one is frustrated in life but could have a quest with the small world observed by that individual. It is fourteen years old story when the author tried to pen down his thoughts "In search of truth". The quest of search for the truth was probably around the life style in the metropolitan city, small towns and the villages. The quest was for finding the reason in the degradation of the human values in the advancement against the money value or the incorrectness in this thinking. Knowing that the human mind is the differentiating factor to understand the answer for the present human state the author had to go back to the root level and track down the progress made by human in the mental plane to reach a satisfactory end.

There would be nothing new in the matter but it has been given a different view with certain scientific tooling not to prove any point but to give a belief that the human minus mind is only a matter like any other matter and would follow all the known rules of science where as the mind is a variable which has allowed to evolve the mankind. The process thus described is an attempt to generate a rule that is followed by this variable known as kind. If the historical past allows to postulate the hypothesis the theory allows to indicate the probable routes for the future, which could generate an interest in many for the obvious reason. The theory made is on human values and the logic sense and their role with the developing human and accordingly arriving in a designated mental frame for any unit small or big of individuals, families, social groups, organisations or the nation and further one biggest conglomeration of one mankind. A nation is assumed to be the biggest unit present. This is the main concern and so mental frame of some nations have been explained in details. The human values have shown to progress in a sinusoidal fashion (swings), which could be in a logarithmic progression where as the logic sense movement is in a straight-line fashion. The hypothesis can be a tool for the researchers to divide the peaks and troughs mentioned by the actual age from the history, there is scope of further making subdivisions in the mental frame such that all the existing nations can be placed into the format for evaluation of their status.

PAVAN RAINA

ACKNOWLEDGMENT

My mother has been source for enlightening me and providing the energy in more than one way. She is and always would be more than guru and the source of inspiration to me.

I am indebt to Kirti (my wife) and Tulika (my daughter) who have smilingly shared all the problems and encouraged me to follow the concept of values and prompted me in my search towards aim of human life.

Professor A.K Mukherjee (of Delhi IIT) and Late Dr J L Pandit (Prop. Hill Grove School, Delhi) have been the strongest critics in the initial stage of my writing and allowed to give it a shape.

I am grateful to all my near and dear ones for their lasting impression; their association has left on me. I am grateful to all those known people who had indirectly helped me to evolve the concept.

Thank you.

SUMMARY

The Evolving Human And The Future World is about the development of mankind from a perspective of the evolving mind and the consequent effect. The book has four parts and summary of each part is described here.

Chapter 1 -------------------- "The Swinging Mankind"

The first part "The swinging mankind" informs about the human growth and describes about the values so experienced by the people. It describes the growth of civilisation from the grass root level. The root level is taken as that of animals who only know to survive and live with nature and have the values of purely natural instinct. The growth of the civilisation has been described on the physiological factors that could have emerged after the first breaking of the natural instinct. How the physiological factors in stages have given him the knowledge of certain elements, which were consequently termed as "the values". Certain probable sequence of events have been indicated so as how at various stages knowledge acquired lead to emergence of positive and negative human traits. The chapter informs how living in small groups and sharing at the lowest level could have generated various new sentiments, feelings which they were able to communicate in some form. Further the chapter informs about civilisation has passed through the landmarks of tribes, colonies and nations indicating how each such format was associated with an additional human values.

The first hypothesis indicates that emergence of a core value was necessary for giving a stable format and the first stable format allowed to develop into a more progressive civilisation into higher complex level. Each further stable format of civilisation had added another core value. The hypothesis indicates that only the positive values brought the upliftment in the society and made it move up in the ladder of civilisation and in term of superior human behaviour. It is also indicated how negative traits emerged in the human society causing instability in the existing format and made him reach in a different more complex position generating two distinction branches. One group continuing with positive traits reached another higher stable format generated higher values where as the other group with negative traits delayed their upliftment. Food for body was the most important item even before the civilisation started. The importance of changing habit of the food is described at various levels with respect to the upliftment, which has a direct nearing on his existing state and the survival.

The second hypothesis is that the human civilisation has moved in a sinusoidal* behaviour. The civilisation as come across three peaks till now and one last peak possible remains when either all the people of the world would live a long harmonious life or would make the mankind collapse. Each peak of the curve represents a different stable human format and successive peaks belong to the stable format with bigger human unit. Each peak is followed by a decline, which represents the instability growing in the existing format. It does not mean that entire human community has become negative but is the intermediate period of trial of positive human whose patience and perseverance gives another improved high point in the forward movement of civilisation. The positive traits in the higher civilisation keeps becoming more challenging as the human values starts unfolding to cater much larger segment of human community. Will the ultimate positive remaining trait be able to appease the entire humanity to make one big humanity community and if so which segment of the world has the chance for such an opportunity?

* *Sinusoidal means like sine curve in trigonometry. It is the curve with swing generating peak and trough.*

Chapter 2 -------------- "Logic Sense and The Nature"

From the very first moment the human has acquired a logic sense he is unable to get rid of it even he thought for it. The second part describes about how developing human came across the changed requirements for his survival and how did he cope with it. This chapter describes how a strong man started becoming weaker physically and to compensate the weakness utilised his mind to develop tools for his survival and started becoming stronger mentally. Indication is given how, knowingly or unknowingly, human has changed from a natural (jungle) man to a social animal. It further informs how he is changing towards a synthetic man. The switch over process is described of human who once was dependent on nature which is bountiful is becoming dependent on natural source which is limited.

The change of living standard with time has been described. The chapter deals with the critical scientific developments, which changed the living style altogether and brought the pace in his thinking process. How the higher developed mind worked for conquering the universe in different direction from the depths of the ocean to the galaxies in the sky. The race still continues today. The growth in medical science has been described. It is indicated how with the rise of logic sense or becoming mentally stronger if human invention in medical science was able to reason and find the solution to various disease and illness he came across newer problems to resolve them. The chapter stresses the human (or any living species) body to be the best machine ever made and in scientific world of engineering and medical science human is either trying to duplicate the functioning of part in a machine to perform better than him or working towards the repair the defective body parts to prolong the body functioning like a machine. The chapter warns that with time the human is becoming independent of nature making him synthetic, which is against the natural law and would generate a cause of worry to the mankind.

The logic sense tries to draw a picture of newer generated need of human in the changing civilisation and thus causing various inventions. It describes of the advancement in science and technology for their end application, which should be for a social cause. What the chapter does not say directly but raises an issue is that these inventions have created a material world where the urge of economy tries to supersede the value. The scientific developed materials are generally for the convenience of human but the prime question generated here "Are these material useful to all the humans or a specific breed working for a larger human cause"?

On the other side in medical science if scientists reach a stage where they can change any human body parts and make it re-function. Would the prevention of death be possible, would it be logical and even if taken as the correct step the cost of the art would be exorbitant to cater only few. Even if few beneficiaries were thought to be great achievers in any field their achievements relate to a specific band of time would become obsolete in future. Would it make sense to keep few such human alive by the art?

Chapter 3 ----------------------"The Humanity Element"

The first chapter gives the details how the evolution of mankind generated certain core values. With reference to inter-human relation the chapter shows that similar conflicting or appeasing situation at different stage of advancement of civilisation generated different experience. The mind has been the focus in the growth of civilisation. In the earlier chapter different values of love, respect, moral values have been associated with higher evolved state and with bigger human conglomeration. Humanity element describes if the smallest unit is associated with the basic core value and when the civilisation grows and is associated with another set of value it has been explained how the initial core value remains important and embedded in the system. The tribe is said to be the smallest human unit with a core value of love, the chapter further interpolates the term unit when the smallest unit becomes one self and the relation of human is explained still remains the same. One set of unit thus becomes self, family and the immediate neighbourhood or relatives where as the another set of unit corresponds to tribal format, colonial format, national format where each one unit is seen as one entity comprising of many humans. The unit thus becomes a point of interest, which should have specific sets of values for constant rise in the mental evolution.

The behaviour of molecule and atom around the nuclei in any element is correlated with the human values. If the body minus mind remains a matter with composition of various elements of inorganic and organic nature the matter would follow the rules of physic and chemistry. When the mind comes in the picture the values come in picture. The behaviour of body and mind is explained to follow similar relation but with different variables of our interest.

The theory also indicates how in the process of evolution we have started from a smallest unit of self, moved to make the unit bigger and bigger one. The chapter indicates the trend when we are proceeding towards the stage which would require to make the biggest unit possible "Humanity" or could disintegrate all the formations back to square one to the original state.

Chapter 4 -- "Future World and the Mental Frame"

The human have been in the quest of something they do not possess physically, be in engineering, medicine or any social science area. Similar things apply for the larger units of tribal, colonial or national format, which have been our tools for the describing the progress of civilisation. In material what we donot possess comes out by dreaming the best technique available in nature for example bird flying in the sky could have generated the urge to make the aeroplane. The similarity of mind has been utilised in devising the computers and the software driven technologies. Similarly on the non-material side the quest for unknown keeps working. The author has tried to give an end as a common factor, which one can dream today and forms a useful basis in the present context.

The Mental frame chapter is an attempt to utilise the tools of the first three chapters to categorise various units of civilisation described in certain format. These formats belonging to different stage of growth has similar end requirements but the paths to achieve are different. The subject tries to indicate different paths for them, which has larger significance in the present world. In our theory we have considered the national format to be the largest unit existing on the day and thus various countries big and small have been considered for our point of view of the discussion.

It would be interesting to note that many nations we have today do not come at all in the national frame. The end goal knowingly or unknowingly being the same generates few proposition of short cut in the much aware world of today. The positive and negative traits come in picture here as the short cut to both the positive and negative traits are there one could follow. It is simpler to follow short cut in negative traits where short cut in positive traits would require higher human values than existing in that part of the system. Individual countries have been discussed in details with reference to their existing mental frames so devised by the theory and relation of their policies and doing that could affect them or the world.

INTRODUCTION

We humans are fortunate to be born in the advanced stage of the evolution but are we advanced enough to be proud of our deeds? The answer could be NO. The evolution must have taken thousands of years to reach where we are but there are equal forces being applied to diminish all the good work. But that too is also not as simple as we have enough good minds to work towards it which is a design of a superpower which the majority today make try to overlook. "Evolving............" is the story of human mind as it could have behaved, in the early stage of human evolution. It has been tried to explain how the evolution of mind could have generated knowledge about himself and the as a consequence what all he did and achieved as a land mark known to us. The story tries to explains inter relations between the human in different stage which tend to become complex with advancement. Each one of us would have some knowledge of habitat today in a very rich country, very poor country, a remote village, an advanced village and so on. The knowledge could be correct or incorrect or partial, one could have acquired knowledge through book, in school, by people or by any other media. The knowledge cannot be wrong or right as what ever one knows could surely exist somewhere in our world even if it does appear to look irrelevant as we go by the facts which are projected. At least all good things are not necessarily projected to the extent as they do not form attractive news to the general mass and thus not influence them.

On the other hand there would be a good amount of people who are specifically aware of habitat of different region not because they have visited but because they have been working with them and have come from advanced wealthy world and are dedicating their life for the needy ones in their country or else. For such people country is no barrier and see human as human wherever they be situated. Such people would never require any recognition as they are busy it their good job which is self-satisfying.

Awareness is an intermediate state of mind where upon the knowledge gained one tries to apply the skill which happens to be either constructive or destructive in nature. One applying he skills in a constructive way could make reach towards realisation which is self satisfying and full of contentment. There is another state where awareness is utilised in exploiting other for selfish gain. Section applying such skill would mistake themselves as intelligent for a simple reason they possess to project and win the gain from a short term perspective but leave a mark in the society which has a long lasting negative influence. Through out the world such negative influencing sections are working and more known which does not require a self discipline and an easy path to follow.

By knowledge and his skills the potter is able to carve the earthen vases which find its place in the home of people for decorating with flowers and generating a harmonious atmosphere, though physically that make himself satisfied for a moment at least. A dedicated potter could be more satisfied with lesser knowledge than the section using it who could be having more knowledge but using the skills with a selfish end. Selfishness is an attitude which could not be eradicated in a larger point of view. One established stable country could have selfishness as a motive to keep his countrymen happy as a necessary tool and could be affecting the other part of the world which does not have a direct impact to them in a short term strategy but could be seen hitting back with time in some other form. One prominent section today is of terrorist who are aware that they would die in the process but create all sorts of fear in the world. What they lack is the core value of love within them and have been influenced by the society deprived of positive values. Such skill is of no use if it only takes them further away from the world of realisation. Realisation word is used because it is the source for experiencing pain or pleasure in the human mind and the source of happiness, the source of satisfaction, the source of contentment which any way they would be searching in a wrong way and ending up in causing misery.

The four words used as knowledge, awareness, skill and realisation are the very basic tools of the management of any level. Do we all understand the difference? Awareness can be understood when the knowledge gained is used which could be of negative or positive in nature. Human in complete awareness and with positive skills can have a long lasting affect on the society and we do see such individuals working day and night. But in the present format of the world divided in different name of countries with different developed religion and culture in their society there is lot to give and take for balancing the act as basic requirements remains the same for any human of any part of the world.

Let us see the simple difference between these words and take an example of one of the thing which came in human knowledge in the very beginning, it is flame. All have the knowledge that it is dangerous and can burn. There is also awareness about it and thus is handled with caution. It is the skill used in positive way that has allowed him to use it for cooking the food to extracting the metals from the ore. The knowledge of flame and heat also makes aware that it is one of the essential ingredients of our body which keeps us energise but how many of them reach to the realisation level. If one has realisation one would be able to correlate the flame in the body and the flame in the mind which is as destructive and also as constructive as we know and which is so near to us that we may not require to go the external burning fire for its realisation. This is to say that

1. For realisation one need not wander many places but could be experienced from the closest that is self.
2. It has a positive effect and influences the surrounding and
3. Requires a great effort in one which keeps becoming more and more difficult to bring in the system when the unit increases in size as family or a society.

The first chapter is on the values. The focus is given on the core values which have been the cause for the inter-bonding between them. For instance we would see that love has been the primary and most important value ever generated to start the society formation of smallest level. In fact there is only one value love that exists and would continue to exist. As the human society grew and developed in different format the requirement of love also started growing which gave a different set of names such as respect, moral value and humanity. As mind has been free to wander any positive growth has equally generated a negative aspect and so is the case with values. The values at time become debatable issue among people when the negative branches are also brought along with the topic. The negative aspect also is a part of the growth in the civilisation but not the cause of the growth.

The negative values thus have been focused such as comparison, jealousy etc which could have only delayed the process of evolving but does not find place in the growth pattern. As the core value love starts shaping into another value respect in a larger group the negative values also multiply with more people and more mind to react. To combat the negative aspect positive force is required and it is not the quantity but the quality that wins over it. Even if the negative force is more in quantity or with the number of human there would be a positive force generated from some quarter and would influence for the growth and the reason we still evolving.

The knowledge gained in each step has generated positive and negative aspects. It is further described how only the positive values have made the evolution move forward. It is described how and why positive values resulted bonding within the different units of growing human society. The further describes that once a stable society is accepted negative values start surfacing out. After a length of time even if negative values cause disharmony in the existing society it does mean that another positive value is required in another form of society to give a stable form. Our present mankind has passed through the troughs and crests (ups and down) and has resulted to reach the present stage of (mental) evolution. The trend allows to make a hypothesis which could be extrapolated so that the intelligent people today can take precautionary measure for a peaceful co existence of our children and great grand children.

The first chapter thus informs how the tiniest knowledge in human generated the basics growth of the mind and how the values thus were recognised and adopted as a stable living pattern. We would see that the basic value described is love and it also goes with the period when the basic *knowledge* was being acquired from no knowledge zone when we start calling them a developed human being. Initial period of gaining the knowledge thus had the widest time span before the negative values emerge to counter the growth. The second important value mentioned is respect was acknowledged with more developed human. This was the stage where human were *aware* for the basic requirements which they had learnt and experienced down the generations. But as the mind gates were already opened it was on the growing path with addition of newer knowledge. Similarly the third value found was 'moral value' where we exist and this stage coincides with the *skills* application for to influence the human. Today we observe skills and anti skills being used by the different section of the world which could be appearing at the height of development and also at the height of fear on the existence of mankind. We have to cross over this hurdle sooner or later and are in the midst in identifying another set of parameter to bind us which is humanity. Humanity could lead the world to the stage of realisation in that sequence, but would we reach the realisation state at all?

We shall find out.

The second chapter is devoted to another aspect which had come out due to the positive thinking of developing human mind which is termed as logic sense. This chapter is easy to understand as it deals with the scientific growth that all are well versed. The chapter describes the sequence of newer need and consequent newer development to what ever the human were able to dream. With growing mind physical activity was reducing and thus the reference of comfort was also changing and thus newer invention for newer needs have been pouring by the scientist. The scientific development was on the basis of hypothesising a dream and then working towards with justification to convert into usable function. The function varied from inventing medicines to developing satellites. One thing has been limited till now is that the biggest invention had the limitation of physical nature. The logic sense being part of human being cannot escape from the negative portion and thus the development for the destruction was not left behind even though it could have been invented for the cause of saving humanity.

It has been the human mind that is evolving as that is only one way track once it has come out from its natural state. If the values were generated to redefine their living in harmony at different stages it did not have any place for proving anything. When justification type of notions which emerged from logic sense were utilised to compare with others for the sake of showing their superiority it added complexity within inter human community disturbing the harmony and resisting the positive growth.

Growth forward is unquestionable as that is a natural recourse by the powerful God whose flawless design does not have a slightest snag and has to end in meeting him. It is our ignorance that in assuming our self most knowledgeable and intelligent we are trying to compete with each other and at times even trying to attack the humanity but any such desire would eventually fail and the human mind would step forward with more challenges ahead.

If we see over the national boundaries and above the man made religion and cultures the growing network of technology has allowed the knowledge to flow anywhere very easily but ultimately we are dividing the world into two halves. One half enjoying the pleasures of all kind where as the other half living in all sorts of deprived conditions. The free information and knowledge available does not speak about it. These two halves are beyond the limit of any specific nations and exist through out the world in different proportions. The deprived ones are sacrificing their life for the pleasure of the other part without their knowledge. There are great many organisations and individuals who are working for their up-liftment without being in the news and limelight but more than that is required at present. The pleasure of one part has to reduce the sacrifice of other and so give and take for human by the human could only solve the riddle. There are two routes to reach such place either by achieving realisation through knowledge and adopting universal skills or wait for anti skill for destruction in his awareness. For the benefit of our brothers, sisters or children or grand children let us keep away the second option.

CHAPTER 1

THE SWINGING MANKIND

Man The Superior Animal

The man is the most superior animal existing but it is not enough to be happy and proud to be about it. It is millions of years we have reached the present stage and time to analyse the simple steps that has allowed us to reach this advanced stage. Have we only gained in the process or have we lost something also. Introspection in the matter may allow us to understand and give a chance to think whether we could be able to survive the development.

Survival is the natural instinct of every living species. We have disintegrated the species by their different habitat developed with time as animals roaming on the land, aquatic creature living in the water and the birds. There are also different bands of creature on the land, which are of smaller size nevertheless not weak. Microorganism and bacteria's are another variety of species, which are not necessarily seen as the other ones but are equally important in its existence and the existence of our universe. Each of them has unique way for their survival. For our discussion let us leave the microorganism and rest we divide between man and animal.

Not separating any, all follow the same the natural cycle-after birth are guided by parents for their security till they become independent to face the world before them. They have sex instinct to reproduce to perpetuate the race and ultimately die leaving the physical body behind with no meaning in it. The instinct of self-survival gives the rise to the basic need of the food. Man or animal eats their food and leaves rest for its body to do the function for processing. The very fact that man understands the value of this body mechanism makes him different and superior. The developed man is able to correlate the inputs required giving them terms as vitamins, proteins, starch, carbohydrate etc and further relate it with the taste. The importance can be understood from the fact that the stomach accepts the food consumed and does the processing as required but the developed man is equally concerned for the little tongue for the taste that is consumed. The food without any taste and with all the nourishment required cannot be accepted by it except for once for trial or for the people who are under doctors order for their part of not respecting their own bodily requirement in some part of their living. It is assumed that animals may have the sense of taste but it is not an important one. This clearly distinguishes animal from the man. Food is the primary source of energy for survival but what is, that which is changing the habit or selectivity of it, the very fact that we are able to term it, as the basic need does not make us great or superior. Why we compare ourselves with animals? Are they worst lot on the earth? Definitely not! It is a pity that we easily compare man with animals and at odd cases assume to be worst than animal. But we do not have any right to compare with an innocent creature who at all is not bothered to relate one self with the man.

It is the brain, which comes in the forefront, which may be the culprit in thinking so. In fact the thinking source is brain and one singular part that separate us from the rest. This thinking power of a man, which clearly separates from the other species, is of so basic in nature that a person with no formal education could understand. Let us go in the age millions year back when the man was another animal in the world and living in the natural way like others and find the probable sequence of the development.

Formation Of Tribes

Making Of Mankind

The brain is the separating factor of a man from animal. Lets find out how the early civilization could have been seeded and came into existence. Lets go the stage when man and animal were species living in their own spheres of jungle. The basic natural instincts for survival were same. Man because of walking on two legs and having two hands free for any action would have been the primary reason for the development. With variety of food available as fruit, vegetables, flesh he had a better sense of taste and wished to have the food of choice rather than chance. He had two hands free to pluck the fruits and keep the animals at a stones throw. Accidentally using a sharp stone made him realise to use the tools for killing the animals as well as to reach for any fruits with ease. He had a brain as other animals but was struck here for the early seeding in it and thus he had a reason to be proud of being braver than the mightiest animal, which led to draw a comparative line between man and animal. Gradually he developed a variety of tools of odd shapes with available natural options and he acquired the skills to out smart the other existing creatures. Now he was sure to fulfill his basic need of food of his choice comparatively among fruits, vegetables and flesh.

This would have been the first turning point in the mankind when he had the realization of being superior and then his brain started working in search for an idea to keep himself superior. The urge for a secure life was then cropping up which led him to move in groups for hunting and started living together in small flocks. This was the age when the role of a man and women was not well defined and awareness of senses was also not there. When all the individuals were caring for them selves the stronger one were getting more fed because of their sheer physical power and weaker ones were in difficult situation prompting them for infighting in the group.

This was the time when apart from the natural necessary instincts it was the physical energy which was predominant with a spark of additional brain which in the early stage of civilisation did generate certain emotions and feelings such as fighting or attachment which cultivated in strengthening their communication system.

Once they started moving in groups for hunting and living they started sharing food. Infighting among them was reduced and found themselves more secure from the animals in their vicinity.

Now sharing with their counterpart was not merely for basic need but also to attract the other. The urge of attraction must have been for the fulfilment of the carnal comfort rather than after a struggle for it. Consequently living together and sharing in all the basic necessities they started deriving some pleasure and gradually brought this in a habit. He started nurturing a newborn, caring for new mothers. If his colleagues had gone in search of food for a hunt, some were there in the base camp to look after the child and the mother.

A bond was developing among them selves and a division of the areas of work were coming into shape. Some liked hunting, some plucking fruits and some caring and nursing the weaker ones to their capability. They were identifying their strength and enjoying life with a feeling of more security.

The bond established among them was realised, as *love*, which started becoming stronger with time and gradually it, became a habit or the minimum life requirement. This bond made them sure to meet more challenges in the lighter spirit.

Once the seed was sown in the brain for progress in thinking and he reached this stage he had the new strength to think beyond the worry for the food. Man did something out of the way knowingly or unknowingly, took the risk and found the results fruitful. He developed a sense in his day to day activities and every new though was tried and further its success gave him more fulfilment.

Togetherness was their combined strength, which enabled them to cope the most difficult situation for the basic food and security.

With awareness of more secure feeling and adaptation in the new habitat followed the feeling of love and affection was generated and with generations to follow there were changes in the life style for the improvement and some basic values were being formed.

With abundance of new value realized as love the brain of a man became more intelligent and started using more skilful activities in their daily life style which resulted in forming some definite norms. The distribution of work was made so that instead all chasing to meet their daily food some were made responsible for searching the food while some were given the duty for safeguarding the infants and nursing mothers from the unknown environment.

With confidence gained in the new system their food habits changed. May be from a natural forest fire they found baked vegetable or flesh which tasted better and gradually found the art of cooking their food in fire. The man must have found that baked or roasted the food was palatable to eat and also easy for digestion. Such acts brought wonder in their life style and even may have been instrumental for discovering the technique to generate the fire by striking two stones. He must surely be thrilled by the achievement and this was the reason to feel happy about it. The changing food habit must have been the first step to get away from the jungle and the habits that they followed lead them in formation of tribes. In fact this was the time that they invented the mind and the potential of wonders that it can perform.

Let us analyse their mental process in the changed environment.

The animals primarily live in a natural circuit following the basic rules for survival and natural instincts. The energy utilised by them is chiefly in physical in nature. The developed human now had a small portion of mind developed which was different from the brain of animal. The energy used though was predominantly physical in nature there was a small utilisation of mental energy which was different. Though the requirement for living remain the same for food, shelter and procreate the opening of mind and using the new mental energy was fun in all the related activities.

Living in pockets made them feel more sure for their basic need of food and security (which is a mental state) thus gave them the opportunity to tap the skills connected to their daily activities.

It was their hands, their legs, their voice and the natural resource available in abundance (trees and plantation) which were used as the tools in their aid for improved living. Hunting had become simpler with sharper tools, three branches and leave made a better shelter along with the addition of joy due to cohesive living. Though this joy felt was a mental feeling very new to them was enough to activate through the physical action such as running (using legs), swinging (using hands), and shouting (using voice at high pitch). It was their physical organs which they could have used in a different manner to give newer meaning.

Nevertheless all this was not so simple to be done by few persons alone. Living for individuals survival to living in groups would itself mean curbing certain one own instinct, and for that reason there were obstacles on the path at every point. In the tribal sections that overcame the initial problem had formed certain discipline there were certain people that had time to use their skills in easing out life style by inventing some small useful steps to make their life more comfortable.

Knowledge And Sense Of Disharmony

The formation of tribes had led in setting of some basic norms and the rules for living. The mind was being exploited in this situation to give them more sense of comfort in the group living. They wanted to satisfy every one, they wanted togetherness to continue, and they loved the attachment a wanted to be loved by all of the members. A positive approach for a good cause had been the drive to reach this stage. In this style of living and with some set pattern to be followed there were certain things that were assumed or granted to be followed in different segments which could have been the reason to grow a negative sense some where causing a sense of disharmony in certain section.

Let us consider one event that could have been to surface out the negative element in the mind. The formation of tribe era was responsible to surface out the primary core value of love. This also cultivated the sense of attachment. Love and attachment of man v/s man, man v/s woman and woman v/s woman were the key ingredient in its stability and there were certain things taken for granted till now to fulfill it but let us consider a case below-

A man gone for searching the food for their group made a very big hunt or found some thing extraordinary may be a better knowledge of stones that would ignite a big flame by a gentle strike. Returning home he assumed to get a big appreciation and a warm welcome. May be he was appreciated by many but not by the person he loved more. In fact for the beloved the great act that he wasn't that a big achievement and so did not show a great enthusiasm as much as he expected. There was a jolt in his sense of pride. His imagination started rolling in the other direction. Instead of the motivation for a better achievement the question was raised within him to discover 'why was he not admired by his most beloved one(s)'

We find emotions and sentiments surfacing out in human. Emotions are not necessarily bad. But at the stage where attachment and harmony in life style had given, them the opportunity to assume certain proceeding which activated them in doing new wonders they also had made a reference of happiness, which they would get in return. Making a reference point for happiness and not getting it for any reason gave a chance to think that they would be wrong in certain assumptions and was a point of worry for some.

Let us take another example for clarity-

A man made a big hunt and is expecting a big hug by his folk at home and a big feast. Adding further he thought his beloved one would hug and give him a kiss and they would roll in love for that matter.

Let us see the situation at his home. His beloved had already prepared a feast for her own good reasons but for some reason spoilt it and had to throw at may be one of her child had hit another and created a chaos and spoilt her mood.

He is coming back with highest spirits and she has lost her normal spirit for different reasons what happens when they meet is the universal truth-

Any matter flows from the higher gradient to the lower one Man in higher spirit comes down where, as woman with lost spirit is better. There is a clash in oneself and fails to know what has happened. One feels his sentiments are hurt where as they were not actually except of such circumstances that happened unknowingly.

Opening of the gates of brain he now had the knowledge of sentiments and emotions. Faint knowledge of emotions led him also to realize as hurt in the above case. To some the hurt emotions became a tool to play as in the following case-

A man who is an achiever for new ideas and development is liked and pampered by his fellow persons around him. But there is one next door neighbour who is keeping a watch on all the applauds his friend is getting. He thinks he cannot contribute in the great ideas as his friend and starts felling insecure. He starts comparing his friends happiness which he is not getting and discovers a method to please himself. If he cannot be an achiever and be appreciated by his friends he can definitely try to defame and make him guilty and feel himself elevated.

This must have been a tricky situation and this sort of pleasure derivation was the evil force coming up but was still part of the development of society.

Formation of colonies

Emerging Of Leadership Instinct

As the man had crossed the primary survival natural instinct by his positive efforts there was harmony prevailing in the group following the basic first value developed and also following the living parameters they have developed in the process. But after once the ports of the brain were opened there was no way to go backwards. In the same area with the development when he came across the feelings of emotions and sentiments, expectation and comparison he developed the knowledge of jealousy and was the root cause of disharmony. What it led to, let us see further-

A person who failed or who thought to be failed in one specific area (in technical development in the case above) did not think himself in a hopeless or lost condition but prepared himself to analyse his weakness and strength. He was different from thousands other who has similar thinking of failing to do achievement and reason to be depressed but failed further to apply a cause or lived simply in the superficial harmony around them and were lost in the crowd unknown to anybody, infact unknown to oneself.

What has unpleasant derivation of pleasure led to?

He blames and defames others in a group where harmony is prevailing. There were many such failing people and remained silent and accepted the situation and thus blocked their path to the progress. The motivation energy behind what ever were able to think and do had been in ramshackle.

The hero in the context who simply did not agree with the situation was ready to fight with it. What did he achieve? As he tries to disturb the harmony, people around get agitated, he is asked to leave the group, resistance is there, some verbal and physical fighting is there and the enemy in oneself comes out. He is in crises and has to act to prove himself.

In the harsh treatment, which he is awarded, there are unmotivated failed lot in the section who generate sympathy towards him. Seeing a definite group of sympathizers he finds the strength in the crises. He praises them and asks them to follow elsewhere beyond this territory to live in peace.

The building of new group had emerged because of a bold step taken by one. He is now obeyed and respected by all the followers. He was a leader and if he failed in the beginning now he had a reason for satisfaction. He got what he was searching; his strength was engineering the human mind, which had made him a successful leader. The person withstood the crises and came out with hidden quality, which must have been prevailing but unknown earlier.

In this situation if the first fraction had observed and realized the strength of the person they had thrown out of their group the former must have tried to compromise to make them join hands the self made leader had given birth to an additional knowledge of ego which did not allow it to happen. The new group established itself in a different place to bring back the harmony among its members at the first place and then started adding the skills for the further improvement in the life style. Their basic need of food clothes and shelter remained the same followed by an urge to reproduce and in the gradual process they created their own world.

Ruling The Territory And The Kingdom

The leadership property generated in the development of the mankind was found to be useful skill to govern a larger fraction of people spread in a specific area. Groups which had taken shape and formed a definite society were expanding in numbers and thus area. They had to compete with other groups which were shaping from the fractions of some developing group or upcoming new groups. In such a scenario a native group headed by their leader occupying a territory became a significant for all concerned. The leaders had faithful followers and commanded respect because of the situation and it became duty for the leader to see their return in return. It was clear that the survival of their race was foremost important and their basic need and the security occupied the top most priority. In the changed situation addition of developing skills became equally important. With the aim of living and maintaining harmony in the developing pattern of the society guarding themselves or the defined area became a requirement.

It was the knowledge of respect, which had evolved. The people in this larger group enjoyed utilizing the newfound tool of respect. The leader divided different segment for different area of operation for day to day work and the faith between them was the motivator to do wonders in the movement ahead. The faith, the trust between the leader and his follower was so much that they were even ready to sacrifice their life on the order of the leader as his instruction as it was for the larger benefit for the entire society or colonies.

These colonies must have been formed around the rivers and lakes so that water is within their easy reach. The developed society started utilizing natural resources in their daily living. The wood was used fire, making the huts and the tools. Their food habits were reformed and changed drastically by this time. Definite art of cooking was known and they had identified cereals, pulses, vegetables and fruits. They use to care for such plants and tress and grew them. They were selective for flesh eating with a definite way of cooking that could be digested easily.

The leader of each group or colony formed was able to bring satisfaction in the people by motivating them to work. New development was shaping fast giving and secured feeling was prevailing all around. The leader was satisfied for fulfilling his duty towards the people and people were pleased in adopting and accepting the modified way of living.

Farming became the important profession and that lead to increase enormous knowledge in it. The crops best in that area were ear marked, grown, watered and on harvest time they celebrated the occasion. If hunting had reduced the people had knowledge to command any animal and utilize their specific strengths. They started taming different animals for different application. They found these animals to be very useful once they were given their share of food. Cows, buffaloes, goats, dogs, horses and even elephants were tamed. If cows and buffaloes were the milk producers shared by all, the leader liked to tame elephant to keep him-self on the top.

Awareness of Respect

The colonies were expanding. Population was increasing and with demand development was also coming in practice. The leaders role was now not merely to motivate a small group as in the beginning but was also to ensure that each activity carried out for the betterment by his people does not find any hindrance. This led to the formation of small pockets of different activities and he guided each group for their progress. If one group was busy in farming and another in building houses each group were given charge to put their effort in their specified area to utilise their skills and bring the improvement. The leader had to device a method to interface where the fruits of the labour of different section are shared by larger sections of that colony. A group was made ready to safeguard the territory of the colonies and the people from unknown environment which gave them the feeling of security and carried out their tasks religiously.

The leader was termed as a king whose foremost necessity was to see that harmony exists among the people. Assuring all with the basic need of the food, a shelter to stay and the safety were the key components for keeping the harmony. The working area distinctly had emerged as farming and non farming one and to meet the basic demand of basic need in the people distribution of goods was brought into practice and for every one's convenience currency was brought into picture as a measure of exchange from one to another.

Gradually a social system was coming into shape where the king was ruler and setting the norms to keep the harmony in all the respective sections of farming and non farming which were contributing to the growth of their kingdom. The king had to keep in mind about the welfare of all his people and in turn the people had complete faith in his guidance and thought him to be competent and important for his part of the duty. We would find a tremendous difference in the new kingdom format developed to that of tribal format which was the starting point of development. The food habits were reformed, living habits were changed and improvements in emerging society were the key areas. With every section of farming and non-farming one getting their share for fulfilling their basic need they loved their leader. The people had developed a great sense of *respect* with the leader. The mutual respect between the leader and the people made them to follow some discipline which was the initiating point for various inventions then. Development was observed fast in all the areas of operation. Various tools were developed to help in agricultural side in growing, sowing and harvesting. The physical power was transmitted into animal power. Animals were exclusively tamed for fed for their part of job. Transportation and long distance were done by the animal power as well. Gradually the concept or invention of wheel and the lever helped them to draw water from deep well with much ease. All such inventions enriched the values formed in the mankind at that time and the harmony exists in the early era of colonization.

Attack on Respect

In this era of colonization a definite family set was developed where the basic ingredient of love prevailed which was the nucleus of the growth. A step further out of their homes the same value of love in different groups working in different activities under a common head for the benefit of all changed into the respect which prevailed as unsaid binding in each other. These people had all the reason to be contended as their basic needs were fulfilled. In the stable period groups of people were able to devote in their duties in a realization state and the skills were tapped in development in all day to day activities. The achiever group was satisfied in the achievements and the benefiting groups were satisfied in using newer modes in the work. From the tribal format different groups had come out and formed different colonies and the skills were shaping with different degrees of growth.

The fractions that emerged out in the process in the formation of early colony were two distinctive types of groups. The positive and constructive groups were definitely leading the progress in skills but there were also colony formed out of negative achiever. These groups had the stronger leadership and administrative qualities but lacked the technical skilled achiever in comparison the other set. If an achiever were improving their life style faster, the other colony which was less progressive and lacked in the life style had something to compare, feel jealous and find an easier an faster solution to address the problem. As they had more administrative skills and the ruler saw that their own achievers were immature in comparison to the other colony and knew that they would lag in the progress unless the skills are tapped from the existing source elsewhere. They started the war to conquer the area to steal the craftsman in the peaceful zone.

When the peace was disturbed both the groups had to bother for the basic need and security. The skilled craftsman who have to worry of the basic need and security to work in the state of realisation were disturbed mentally and stronger administrative group found the opportunity to grab the people by showing tem better conditions of basic need and security to be available. This was the step of attack on the harmony prevailing and the attack on the respect prevailing in that era of evolution.

Formation of Nation

The phenomenon of this civilization was spreading in the world gradually and at this stage the entire world the values set were at different points of evolution till now. The continents and islands which were isolated and not in easy access with the major land were linked by the inventions of boats and subsequently ships. In such area civilization was seen at a lower stage (of tribal one) or at places it was one step backward. Finding such state of civilization existing made the colonized people realized their superiority and saw a pleasure in upgrading and teaching them the basic values.

The colonies were generated by the (positive) achievers and (negative) leaders. The positive achievers were the persons who had the satisfaction in trying to educate the meaning of life and a meaningful life. The colonies generated by negative leadership instinct people had something to compare their superiority. Such people being stronger in administrative sense thought to possess the territory to expand the boundary. The vales of mankind set were in a disturbed situation. The situation prompted to make a leader from an achiever group to think for the welfare of the human by in large keeping the values of love bond in the family and the respect generated in the colonization and curbing the anti-tactics generated of the revolting group.

Amalgation of people of different colonies of like-minded thinking gave the opportunity to redefine the territory forming a nation. A nation or state was the area which had definite boundaries to safe guard to possess the peace that was missing. One such nation or state had people with different state of progress of mankind. Tribal era which was termed as the earlier culture among developed section prevailed, culture of colonization was certainly existing and all intermediate minor steps of progress also existed. Redefining the changed values in this developed society a definite family set was there with relation to man-woman-children and sharing of love among themselves was the strength in the first stage. To flourish the custom many traditions and festivals were developed. If the entire tribal era had invented the sense of love it was squeezed into one family which was the guiding factor for the progress in the mankind development.

In colonization with different group working on different activities a sense of social togetherness had developed. The respect value thus generated here was the term used beyond the family which in group gave them the strength to work for the development and move ahead.

The colonization set was also on the crossroad. The values of mankind which wee set at a higher altitude was at stake and the ruler in this turbulent era had started demanding respect to rule as per their wish rather than commanding respect. Such a situation forced to amalgate many like minded colonies to form a nation and simultaneously thought of norms to rule where something more than respect was needed to command more aware and skilled lot of people. A family rule of king was not possible and so the head of nation was formed by the causes of people. To carry out various functions in each sphere certain norms were formed in the shape of constitution. These norms were nothing new but a guideline to be followed by all to form a discipline. It was the emergence of moral value to be followed. The nations following such ethics had succeeded in finding the stability. The moral value was thus the next value generated for the need of that hour above the value of respect.

Today the world is on either side of this area and for finding what next let us first summarise the development till now.

The Swinging Mankind

In Fig. 1.1, the development of mankind till now has gone through the following landmarks. Here we refer the progress with reference to the basic values that were known and nurtured and by the sections of people (positive and the

FIGURE 1.1

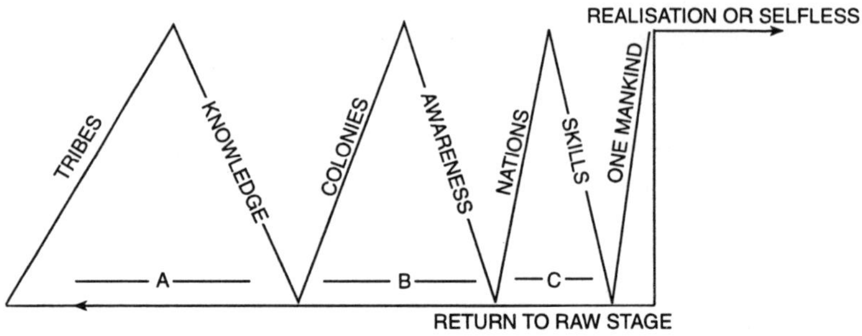

negative) who had the contribution in the evolution of the mankind. The three different areas we have observed are,

1- Tribal,

2- Colonization and

3- National system

The development pattern from the root has followed a definite sinusoidal curve. The peaks of the curve are the regions where the man had generated certain values useful for them to stay in harmony and found some stability in the life style. This was followed by the decline in the process of evolution when the values generated then were not enough to bind losing the acquired stability. It was another set of value that was brought in knowledge and practice to reach the second peak and the stability. Similarly the decline of second peak was there to generate the upward slope for the third peak.

Today we stand here below the third peak as a whole world. Different parts are in the different state of evolution around it. One more peak, the world would be one to share the happiness and sorrow with each other or a bad repercussion could be also a collapse of mankind when one man does not treat another as a human which could destroy the existence of the man himself.

The graphical representation shows that the development of mankind was associated with core values which we have touched in the text. It was the development of human mind as well, which was understanding more about himself. The negative and positive what we call today could be new knowledge because of the changing system. There were also minor positive and negative values generated due to the situation which had the contribution in the process. Let us analyse the progress with such core and minor values with the graphical representation.

The first rise

The first significant development understood the combined strength which generated love (as core value) and affection among them. Sharing of basic need gave them the sense of sharing responsibilities and allowed to cement the basic values in them.

How would have the development proceeded from here? In the new changed state the people must have felt so secured and contended and could not think of development when in their knowledge there was not the sense of comparison. In the early tribal format era there was nothing much to compare in their life style and what they had was only one step backward which was the jungle rule.

"Any development from the natural state if contributes a positive point, there lies a negative point as well".

In the tribal format people started living in groups and started sharing the responsibilities and collectively were stronger to the other natural forces to safeguard themselves but this step would have made them weaker to withstand the external threat individually. To compensate the loss the need arose and forced him to make sharp tools to defend from the animals. In such system small pockets of people comprising of many family members and their children were there as a unit. The day's work was distributed such that some went for finding the food and hunting some cared the safety of woman and the children. Their daily botheration for the basic need must have reduced which pressurized the developing brain for something else. This something else thought could have been around the subject of their food and living habitat and the safety closer to requirement of the natural instincts. On adjusting and readjusting with generations they had adopted to live in small groups which could be controlled. This was the period when mankind had touched the first peak of stability and had acquired the basic understanding and their ability to conquer fear over existing species and had set the basic values of life and where love was the core bonding force among them.

The tribal format gave them the knowledge for added comfort in their life style but with generations and with increasing population in that group and the opening of the mind there were the new positive and negative generation of skills. The positive emotions were evolved from the core value of love. Those who were aware of it at this stage were contributing in creating a stronger bond by working for common goal as nurturing a family and neighbours, developing skills in farming for improvement for the living etc. There were people with negative skill generations also. The negative skills could have been developed by the section who were above the fear of basic need but improper diversion of developing mind at this stages or by a section which was not that sure of the basic needs for some reason. This section instead generated the knowledge of certain emotional values such as comparison, jealousy that were disturbing in nature and leading to the first downward swing.

The leader of the colony who was not ready or organized to answer the new knowledge of such traits saw the existing peace breaking. There were colonies which continue to stay peaceful where as there others were disturbed. The progress in terms of ethic, and life style was among them and counter productive negative option was also there. The growing mind at this stage of evolution was not actually aware what would satisfy them and so the existing leader did not had the capability of control.

The time span covering first rise and the fall marked as 'A' in the figure 1.1 was widest because the human started from rock bottom and were in the process of acquiring knowledge through their physical senses. The easiest knowledge that could be probed was through their organs, through the nature and they found pleasure in the new knowledge they got from what they saw by their eyes, their ears heard, hands and legs helped in doing the experiments. It was the knowledge of taste by the tongue which has a direct relation with the food as the basic need. The knowledge from the nature the tress, bushes, knowledge of surrounding could be weather, cold, hot condition, starts, sun and the moon. Each one of such thing was enough to trigger the mind and find the use in their new meaning in the survival method.

If the LOVE component was the value identified the new knowledge had enough for constructive thinking to meet their basic demand of food and shelter. Growth of manual power or further animal power to enhance their living style was satisfying for the reason

1. That all gave them additional newer knowledge for small modifications. For example staying near water source and watering plants mechanically if required and ensuring the crop grow, knowledge of herbs for their simple ailments etc. All such things were satisfying as it helped their small community and inter relation with love only got stronger.

2. It was the physical energy used without their knowledge in constructive activity that balanced their life to provide the satisfaction.

The strongest negative trait that could have been emerged was only comparison which must have been the start of decline but the force was still not enough to create a strong ripple in the system.

The second rise:

This continued in the downward swing when the people who were aware of the love value and realized its potential to bond till a limit started to know that control of a bigger area, bigger segment of people some thing more is required. Many such colonies were integrated and brought under one territory and headed by a leader known as king. It was the kingdom regime that was responsible for the second rise in the evolution. The leader or the king was certainly with more developed mind at that stage and understood the turmoil and analysed and found the methodology to satisfy the people. What he required was to list out the positive and the negative traits people have generated till that moment, utilize the strength of each, and appreciate them. It was also to provide work to counter people who had negative traits.

It is important to understand that the basic need of food, shelter and reproduce to run the race was the common aim. The value addition taken place was of family system at the primary place and collective working and gathering for the common goal or service for each other. Certain religious ceremonies and festivals were in place for enhancing the bond among them. At work place different work or different type of work were carried out by different section. The different work segregation can be classified by the four segments of Brahmin, Kshatriya, Vanijya and Shudra. These classifications are by Hindu philosophy which tries to classify people with different strengths they possessed to work for a common goal for the unity and harmony for all. The Brahmins were the most learned who were responsible for educating others or guiding the regime. The Kshatriya was next with more of physical strength who were ready to safe guard the defined area as per the instructions of a leader. They were the warriors. Vanijya were the people with responsibility of distribution of necessary commodity to the masses. They were the traders. The last Shudra section was caring of hygiene of the people and necessary cleaning. The hygienic requirements had changed with time. The segregation of these groups were done entirely on the merit of their capabilities where in a big piece of land there were people existing in still different state of evolution. Such un-stated segmentation helped in the productivity and the satisfaction for a larger section of people.

Among the colony leaders probably the higher evolved leader who must have been focusing on the decline of the bond must have been the architect to think one step forward and club few colonies and create a trusted group who would in turn have the reach to the lower rung of people for their requirement and satisfaction. Such trial where there was contribution of many in any decision and in steps to reach the leader was finding an acceptance. His method would have been accepted after a lapse of sufficient time because in such system it was generating another core value as "respect" which was finding the place. Such system gradually with a King ruling a territory comprising of different working segments was developed. This was the time for the second rise of the mankind. Gradual experimentation of the kingdom and upgrading its requirement gave the second peak.

It is necessary to understand that with the evolution of mind at each step there were positive and negative grains generated. If it was the positive grain which was responsible for defining in the living and thinking style and gradually leading to the upward swing of the curve it was the negative grain when became excess were the decline. In such state of the decline the requirement was to combat with stronger positive gain for redefining the philosophy of the mankind. The second higher peak thus was the era of the kingdom regime which was stable period and resulted in many revelations and reforms for the mass.

Such leaders were nurturing their kingdom or territory with their skill in different capacity. The basic requirement were same of basic need and security of the region to maintain peace and harmony. Under the effective leadership each section or the group was working towards the betterment of the entire society and in that process they were awarded by the respect which was necessary for the growth and the results. A person doing laborious or mental job were given the dignity for their contribution as it was towards the common goal. The living standard, eating habits, living habits were changed vastly in this stable period. The processes which were carried out manually or with the use of animal power did find the replacement by all sorts of machine. Mechanization was on rise. Their selectivity for any activity was being narrowed down for better and better. With wide spread increase of knowledge and the skills in all walks of life it was required to spread the skills for the application. The farming was the main source for generation of basic need which was being done by one big segment of people it was the other segment where the knowledgeable scientists were busy developing improvement in the farming process. The scientist were also developing feature to give their life more comfort.

The two sections one utilising physical labour and other with mental labour for the benefit of all was the main source to keep the values intact.

The world was divided in different kingdoms which were quite different and varied in their part of evolution. The development and the positive growth took place in the progressive kingdoms but this improved style of living could have been the cause of disturbance in the less progressive state. There was a king and his commandment one side and the common man on the other end for each other. In the stable state the king commanded the respect from the people and in return the common man got back the trust.

The king who was capable to make the bond not necessarily have passed all the talent to the generation down to keep the trust intact or with the increasing population and the ego of king down the line to increase the territory were the reason for the second down ward swing in the mankind. There could have been other reason also such as between the king and his commandment and the common man there was a gap in the organized set up. There was another section developed in between to balance or let the flow of benefit of either section to the other group. If the former group commanded the respect this intermediate group in absence of real effort demanded the respect. In this period of comparatively more awareness in a certain section the intermediate section which was neither directly linked with the king regime nor were doing any constructive work it was the negative leader ship in them which demanded the respect from the leader (King) and per chance if they did not get it the intermediate section thought to protect their respect and was also one cause that led them for infighting against the ruler.

The span of time marked as 'B' in the figure 1.1 is shorter than the previous one for the reason that the stable human unit became bigger. The system now was not limited to few families but managing a larger human community where there were different sections involved in different task for the common goal to live in harmony. The respect value was the bonding force here as it related in more than one unit of human section. Important to understand here is that

1. The feeling of different sections directly or indirectly interdependent was the force for harmony and the upward swing. The respect was unconditional as they had left on the superior most they though and accepted as king to rule for the administration and monitor the system.

2. The rise of logic sense was sharper as the mechanisation in their work had started. There were enough inventions to reduce the manual work resulting comfort and increase productivity. This era was for the awareness. All those who participated in constructive work in moving the society were the aware lot let it be a farmer, a scientist, a businessman or administrative person.

3. The knowledge in science which works on proof and justification does give realisation to the doers but the non doer in absence of proper knowledge and without being aware were misguiding factor to generate negativity in the system. The word such as justification and proof when applied in inter human relation made a hairline crack in the unconditional love that was there in the tribal system.

4. Farming was not only the source of living but different avenues generated for functioning the system brought a difference in the physical and mental labour that was put for the work. There was disparity generating in the energy put by the person and also disparity growing in the living habitat. Even if people were satisfied in their different living there were negative minds making aware of the disparity to create a rift. The negative values thus generated

created the short cut methods by such section creating mistrust in the harmonious living.

5. If awareness was the cause of second rise by the constructive section more knowledge without proper orientation or half knowledge of another section saw the decline.

The third rise

In such a situation stability of the kingdom colonies were disturbed leading the second decline of the mankind. It weakened the kingdom colonies and their leadership had to think more than prevailing for running the show. Even in the process of evolution today we have all the segments from the oldest unreformed human, tribal colony and the kingdom rule. These sections prevail as a separate unit where human habitat has not reached and also within the enlarged territory of the unit state. Our concern is with the segment that allowed moving further in the step. The disturbing second decline led the higher evolved leader to think further the need of controlling much larger section in a more organised manner. The reach of the leader to the common man had increased in terms of direct contact. The stable period also had given a new shape of living from the various comforts invented. In such a situation of disturbed peace in the existing kingdom colony and there would have been lot of fighting with the adjacent territory kingdoms. This had few advantages such as the leader found a method to oversee the local deficiencies and could allow his people to concentrate on the main issue and his leader ship. The fighting was ultimately the cause of the negative grain of the kings' mind in such a situation. There was no way to go back. Among the victorious king they got now much bigger area to rule. Here a higher evolved leader took the charge to recreate the stability in the form of forming a nation. A bigger chunk of area and ruled with many different kingdoms this area was a mix of a much varied section of people. There were people with different culture from different roots of evolution and so different colonies were nurturing with variations in the life style. The knowledge also had increased and a fancy of a king could not rule the assortment of knowledgeable group and the lower developed section like the tribal era. The result was collective thinking from the learned section and collectively choosing a head the nation who in return had to try to satisfy all the other people of the nation. For carrying out the work a definite moral conduct was formed which the group had to follow. At the core level there was group of leader known as the head of the nation and his associate as ministers. These ministers had sufficient powers that were given different areas of working. These ministers were to make their own plan for the growth. The chain of operation from the head to the common man had become very long. At the core level there had to be law ensuring that the leader and the ministers' work for the benefit of the people and also at the other end with vast difference culture existing to maintain a law and order situation a moral conduct was drafted which was known as constitution. Constitution was drafted in different generating nations and the basis was simple that would work with certain moral value and ethics. *Moral values can not be fixed in general because at any moment to a specific segment the values can be gauged by its own understanding which is not to harm another and it could change with the time and the development.* The "moral conduct" thus was another emerging core value that brought rise in the third swing of the mankind.

In a developed national network at that moment though there were people with diverse culture and diverse stage of evolution it were the more evolved that had the contribution for stability. With the new defined working areas at this stage such as in mushrooming technologies, finances and administrative field along with existing farming, and distribution network which were also reformed had given new life to the nation. Nation building was a new mantra. Considering the learned or more evolved groups they lived in a family which was still nurtured by the core value developed in the tribal era of love. The organization which was a bigger group of operation for the work for the third party which could be a production or management was successfully run by the second core value that was generated in the colonization that of respect. It was the respect between the head of the organization and the working peoples that gave them the daily bread and continued the run the organization smoothly. These organizations which were working for the national interest were now bound by certain moral values which were required to be in place. The constitution serves the purpose between the national leader and his ministers and the common man or the organizations that were there.

The third swing is in the process and thus being explained in depth. The time span shown as 'C' in the figure 1.1 has to be narrower than the previous swing. On one side the human community has evolved in a highly developed stage where as on the other side there are sections which lag very much. In the governing sense it is the national format which is recognised as a stable system. Such stable system has utilised skills in the area of science for human community and also is able to fulfil the desire of the people. Identifying national format as a stable system the world is divided into different countries (with their own historical background) but that does not mean all have reached the same stage of evolution. There are recognised countries which require great amount of support to come near the evolved world but it is the pride or ego which is becoming a barrier. Consequently beyond the national format the world is developing towards the formation of (unrecognised) three different cultures which could be a method for a stable humanity in future.

The third swing

The third swing has importance as it has the relevance with the present and thus has importance to understand certain basic guidelines that prompted us to reach here. The opening of mind to think was the starting point of human evolution from the jungle rule. From here at each step there were positive and negative ideas were emerging out which were responsible for more knowledge in him. It were only the positive ideas that emerged and nurtured by the leaders that lead to the finding of core values to sustain the harmony within an assign group. The positive ideas and its implementation led the mankind to follow the upward swing. The upward swing continued the trend till human were in the process of acquiring the new knowledge, were busy in spreading its message and satisfied. The climax of the satisfaction at least in one defined territory lead to the dulling of mind. The dulling of mind or the lack of new idea led to the growth to the negativity. As the negativity started the dominance, the stable peak was started making a downward trend in the swing.

It should be understood that even if there were the negativity observed in the pockets of the first rise and the mankind development was delayed or reversed that was not of the interest to any one and the one which rose further up was only the meaningful subject.

The first peak generated the value of love bond, which was misused by the negativity, subsequently by generating jealousy and hatred. The positive leaders could do the counter of the negativity by getting larger population in confidence which generated the colonial rule. It was the respect value which was found and nurtured and allowed to attain the second peak. The peak again signified the satisfaction by the mass and dulling of mind and thus loss of new idea. The negativity this time was to attack the value respect that was developed giving the decline trend again. The positive people had to devise the method to change the trend and again they took the same route by increasing their influence in much increased territory or population. This much larger territory was given a name as a nation and the value generated was moral value to hold it as a unit. In each rise or in each developed segment which is of much bigger territory mankind exists which still lags in the race but is again not significant.

The process of development is non-returnable one-way path. The sections of mankind that lags and are behind the race can only blame their destiny. This section does help to awaken certain values which people forget in the developed society. It is work of developed society to lift the underdeveloped and doing so they can find and observe certain core values existing in so called underdeveloped society but they do not understand. Going up the ladder does not mean to forget the past and the known values but to keep the known value intact and adding more of them to suit the new developed situation.

If in the developed nation where core value is moral value from the point of national stability we can observe the importance of other core values which are equally impcrtant in day to day activities. A small unit, be a family, be a small industry can run smoothly only if there is a bond of love within them. The love in a small industry would have a larger meaning of feeding many family and keeping them away from the thought for the basic need. The next stage considering small states in a nation or large industrial sector they are like colonial rule and its sound running upon the trust or the respect within the inter groups of the unit.

FIGURE 1.2

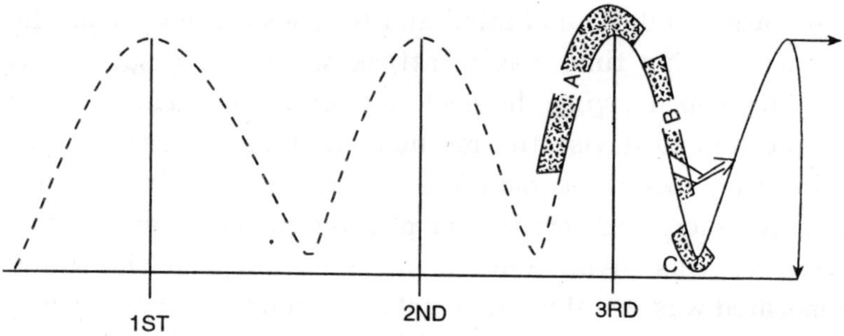

The third swing in detail: As the present mankind is around the third swing we require understanding in more details. Let us discuss on certain topics which relates to the higher positive values which people have worked out due to their shear strength of being superior human.

Development and the state of realisation

Realization may not be understood to the same extent by all but is the state which works on the basis of elimination of self. Realisation is also a state without any end. In any circumstance the state can find the process for the improvement. Realisation is a process which people attain at different state. As one rises higher to the physical requirements his realization is understood to be higher to others but a realized person would see all humans with a similar view. Such noble people when work for a nation formation or national integration they try to work such that in all the sections they are able to bond love, strengthen the trust and teach the moral values.

We can not oversee the fact for the pains of the people who are responsible for the trend to move the family forward, move the society forward, move the country forward and move the mankind forward. If we see the history of a recognized family, a recognized industry or a business house or a nation all of them would have swinging pattern. All have high and low points at different times. Is there any similarity among their behaviour?

Yes if we analyze we would find that only self realized leader is the cause for the high points of any state. Why we call them self realized person? All such leader would have attributes of dynamism, have risk taking attitude, having high moral, are duty and discipline conscious and a posture of confidence. Whatever action they do is for the good of society and not for themselves. Such persons are ideal for making reference as the image of contentment.

Such persons necessarily have to possess a sound and happy family life, educated in a rich culture. Why? The moral values and the discipline in a person is an outcome of deep observation and understanding which starts at home, is schools and society. In the best of these situations available it is only the best opportunity to get proper guideline but it remains entirely to one self to rise above the normal norms to serve the betterment of the larger society, larger national interest and larger mankind.

A child is born in a normal society and gets all the love and affection. His world is only his parents, neighbours and teacher. He grows, marries and has children. His society and the world is changed now. He is able to bring the happiness in his family. Now as a realized great person goes ahead to serve the mass with his leadership instinct. His grooming in a happy family and comfortable and satisfied life thereafter the self motivation of such realized person makes a way to work for the society. He is appreciated, loved and liked by all. Earning fame would not be important for him but his family expands as a large society and is not limited to his family and children. The association of immediate family member with such a realised person only provides an opportunity to straight away see a bigger world and serve the world. Contrary the realisation and association with a larger society would make the physical bond of immediate family weaker if the other members are soaked in materialistic pleasure and so disassociate with such person. Such dedicated individuals are responsible to help in the formation of nations. Forming a nation would mean to rule out the atrocities which people would be facing to make them free and independent.

Realisation and art:

With the progress of mankind there has been a tremendous change in the life style. If in the remotest time the human was totally dependent on his physical activities for survival on his gradually up gradation he started becoming dependent of mind. This change of basic assets in human resulted in the changed requirements for their basic need even such as eating habits. Socially human had formed certain customs, rituals with time and kept upgrading them which as the core helped to form a bond within them. These rituals related to the either births, marriages and deaths which were and still are the critical cross roads in an individual life or related to the God where spiritual force was inducted as a common factor. Development of art at an individual level could be a part playing in social segment but that was able to generate the realization to individual and guide many. The art of music the art of dance the art of drama are of such nature. A classical dance which pleased the people to a dancer it also was able to generate a sense of realization for two reasons. One mastered on his/her physical body or a part of body and the rhythm generated was able to please so many. A singer similarly was the one who was able to attract people and master his body. The wordings of songs were used to sooth the emotions where one was able to link personal life or dream. Such social activities formed a definite culture of the society.

The third peak of the sinusoidal curve with the advancement of technologies such art was further enriched by development of many organs to add the flavour in music and for the reason it was provided to people through the audio system. A good music was able to relax one's mind after the hard work. Hence the peak of the third peak of the mankind development a definite culture was generated that was far beyond the boundaries of caste and religion and had its own developed society and was beyond a national boundary.

The fast culture

The culture was the reason for the decline of the third peak which has lot of bearing with the present time. The technical advancement simultaneously happening around the world had the effect in the culture. The technical advancement made the life of the people faster. The speed of the life of an ordinary person lying at this stage was faster than one could cope with it. In such fast moving world nobody found time for any thing and started finding short cuts to erode the basic values which were embedded till now. Short cut made the people to move towards physical level of needs. The basic values of love, which with time were found to be of mental nature to bond a larger world, became physical. The change of the meaning for the core value was the starting point of degradation of set culture. The Respect as the second core value was commanded by the head of family or the leader of colony or at this stage any organisation as part of the evolution. With the changed attitude the respect found the physical way to command. The rapid technological advancement was also assisting in their process of going physical. The third component of the core value that is moral value also found in fluid state. Moral value which can not have a complete global definition but an attitude with all without any difference was easily at the point of attack. Corruption, cheating or making different set of rules for different people without anybodys consent are the break point.

The section which was busy in the reformation or the development was finding the positive way out for every and any one and such people can understand the importance of associated values such as tolerance, sacrifice and patience as they have to do in their life for the achievement of the goals they have set. The other section which is must bigger in dimensions with the pace started going far from such value and made their life more physical and lonely. The situation in one section helped in demanding the recognition because of the imbalance prevailing in the world and for the commercial gains. Hence in a section of world where there was plenty for the basic need of survival another culture was established.

Beyond the national level accordingly we have three different cultures in place which becomes important for knowing what could be lying ahead.

The three cultures:

(1) The western culture

One section of humans were ahead in the development and among those who were in the nation which were democratically ruled and were liberal (which is a positive path of progress) made in roads of sharp upward trend in scientific improvements which raised the human living style. Comfort was added even if it was not required and which converted in a value. For comfort one had to go for more work, more money and thus speeding the life. It should be understood such place still remains the place for individuals and the groups who dedicate for their life for cause of development. Their development work is for entire human society and it is important for them to have the comfort. They are the thinker and the doers and spent most of the time for the society up gradation and a little time what remains for them selves should have the comfort what they get. They would still understand the meaning of patience and sacrifice, which they would be doing to reach the goal and hence would be realised people. On the other end there were persons who got the comfort as their prime aim and work towards it. These persons were above the problems of basic need and security and their meaning of the life was being compared with standard of living and consequently there was a great damage in the human values.

The western culture where the value of love appears to be reducing at the first place, is trying to find back the real meaning. The love was the primary and most important value in the mankind development. Physical love has its own role to play at time and appropriate place but love generating human-to-human bond had the emotional ingredient which is missing out to a larger extent. It has been overshadowed by the physical love. In absence of emotional love one even opts taming a dog or cat or some other animal because he trusts them more. In the process the absence of trust is also seen in all walks of life. This is not to say that animals should not be loved but not at the cost of human themselves In fact the best situation would be when he rejoins the value and the bond and starts loving the entire nature.

When the life was being compared with standard of living the self cropped up in individuals, groups and the nations. Distortions of husband – wife relation, distortion of child and parent relation are the cause of it. Dishonesty and cheating are the reason for it. Conspiracies and scandals are the result of it. This culture being in the highest region of skills and development are likely to have the intoxication of feeling of being supreme. This is one big hurdle in their path. Any individual may easily come out of this trap but to bring up the entire culture out of the wood would be herculean task and whoever succeeds will be one of the greatest leader of the present times and for the last time in the history.

If we notice at the core of this culture every one is trying to be independent. Be a boy, a girl, man or woman they want to be independent and so the values within them are decreasing. Unaware they are becoming dependent on material or money and are the cause of bringing self at the individual stage. The final achievement would be possible when they realise the dependence of themselves over the material. Defining the essential basic need and minimising the material dependence they could reach the realisation state where in mental happiness rules over the physical. This culture can reach such place as there is nothing impossible, who can do and reach the next higher stage.

As far as which nation or the group of nation can contribute such a noble job would be one which is led democratically as any other form will have a force or a binding on people which itself means the devaluation of the mankind. It would be impossible to achieve such an Herculean task which is not liberal therefore. So in the western culture in the existing state of mankind and scientific development there is a possibility of emergence of a leader in a democratically ruled area, which may guide the world or the entire humanity to give a new dimension of value where there would be more happiness and contentment all around but only if it is able to cope up with the forces emerging in the scientific development area do not make a blunder to perish the man and the mankind itself.

(2) *Eastern Culture*

The second culture existing is lagging behind the former western culture in the graph 1.2 and is marked B. This culture is present in the southern eastern world including countries such as Japan, China, India and neighbouring regions. The people still follow Buddhism and Hindu philosophy here and spirituality could be the cause, which separates us from the western culture. In this culture at the grass root level the values of mankind are still more important. In the process of following western culture we have started observing distorted values similar to the western culture but is limited to certain level of society which is indicating one probability that this culture also would follow the path found by the former which is the easiest of choice but whether the entire culture follows it would be a difficult question. For this reason this culture does exist in the decline of the third swing where as the western culture has already touched the third decline and making an attempt for the rise.

This segment of the world does have more population, it has sub segments, which are lesser, developed in the evolutionary graph, and people living style are in two extremes of poor and rich. All this has a significant contribution in keeping more attached with the spirituality and making follow the life in accordance to the teaching of great spiritual leaders' life Buddha and Krishna and making a separate culture. To a portion of this mixed society the knowledge of the habitat of the former has been accessible giving them a time for evaluating the good and the bad points. Evaluation by the leaders would have impact in totality which could be the guide for good or bad to follow in total or to selectively find out the good points.

The peak of the third swing has been the cause for the sharp achievements in the mankind. The western culture which was able to keep its major population above the basic need saw a sharp development in technological field.

This development which generated a satisfaction in the person directly involved due to his/her dedication in the positive activities gave a material satisfaction to others. The development changed the life style it increased the speed of life to compete with each other and finally a sense of independence has been generated. On the other side the second culture at the peak because of the mix and high population found another area of sharp achievements in their third peak which was human oriented. It was the philosophy which was enriched in different way in different region.

In this stage rich culture was stated to exist only if all the values in the individual and social pockets were alive or further enriched. Stronger human bonds were possible only when positive mental approach was there in them. A man would be ready to die for a good cause of the people is an example of such approach against the social disintegration and individual independence at its height in western culture calls for breaking the law. At this level of western culture a person would like to attain every thing one wants for himself rather than for a common cause that is the phenomena, which tilts the mental behaviour towards physical. If it was the positive mental energy that generated lots of achievement in technology at the peak in the eastern culture the mental positive energy was responsible to generate innovations in arts which have the human bonding implication.

The art was the mental development which incorporated the physical senses and that was the unknown reason to satisfy the flock. Let's take example of songs, dance and the drama. The songs, poems, and dance like things were invented in the colonial time for relaxing the mental strings from the busy schedule. It was the process of relaxing the mental muscles. At the third peak when skills were at the highest level with improvement in music and dance with physical skills or instruments. The art was appreciated when the sequence vibrated the audience mentally. The meaning, the rhythm, the action and the emotions (which were larger than its face value and related to the social conditions) were appreciated by the mass. As this region was nurturing lots of religion which was the outcome of smaller social segment within the national boundary the development of such art helped to nurture the same.

With the advancement of time and the technology the good and bad habitats of different world were known gradually to each other. The western culture with their advancement and with their sense of achieving independence had used this art to derive the pleasure where there was a shift of nature from mental to physical. The songs, music drama started becoming more popular in this segment which tilted the physical sense. Such phenomena also as on the day could be seen making in roads but is limited to one section which tries to compete with the western culture. The third peak of the curve shows the height of skill and equally in this mental status it calls to know and be aware of skills around. The skill of a man here can be said utilised if he can amalgate the strength in development area made of being made without the loss of the values of mankind. The cause of decline after the peak is significantly clear of western culture at the lower end of the curve for striving independence at the individual level. If the selfishness is uprooted they could emerge in the final upward swing of the mankind. In the eastern culture the selfishness has creped in groups and in a section of individuals and is the reason for the decline in the third swing but it has yet not affected the entire culture.

The advantage ahead

If the mankind follows the sinusoidal curve very identically in all the culture the eastern culture will have to follow the path laid out by the western culture and would lag behind all the time and would be guided by them. After the third peak the eastern culture have a distinct advantage to reduce the downward slope at a much higher level for the final swing. The third peak itself is symbolic of wide spread knowledge and its application awareness and a sharp sense of logics for interpreting tomorrows need. It is the peak where human skills can be applied in any direction. The skills and the logics for the positive growth could be the way ahead for guiding the world.

Where does the eastern culture stand today?

And how would it follow?

In the scientific development period the actual pleasure lies in inventing, in utilising and experiencing it. The approach in this region of the swing for improvement of living standard would be strong and similar to what western culture has experienced. With the wide spread knowledge and the skills they have the opportunity to blend the advancement and reduce the weakness from the western culture's experience to give a positive result.

The human value and the scientific development are very lopsided in the eastern culture. The scientific development cannot be stopped inspite of knowing its weakness as it is a path of no return. No development further could only deteriorate and bring to a dead end which is not possible again. Accepatnce of development in a modified way so that the mankind values are taken care of could be one way at the cost of the experience of western culture.

This modified blend may or may not give a new equation directly but it calls for a leadership in a realised state to balance the equation and so they have the opportunity to pause the negative growth in values at the cost of comfort. If the eastern culture has lot to take from the western culture on the development front the former has lot to give in the mankind areas. In the eastern culture the values still in majority of people are deeply imbedded that the downward slope of the sinusoidal curve has to be gradual and a sharp downward trend is not possible. The situation calls for the leadership which straighten the negative direction of declined values. If the western culture has achieved the best in development for their comfort they still lack their satisfaction as the real pleasure person gets from the surrounding and is searching for it. A negative leader of western culture could realise the values of eastern and could try to exploit and shake for deriving one's own pleasure generating from the jealousy but will not be able to uproot the system and which in turn would educate the strength of their values. As in the western culture described earlier in the eastern culture also the nations which would be governed in democratic frame work and with the liberal system can have the power for a positive growth for the mankind ahead. India is the biggest nation which qualifies to keep the culture alive and even develop further.

(3) The developing nation culture

The African subcontinent and the nations around would come in this category. There are nations are yet to touch the third peak of the sinusoidal curve. Human here are yet to come out of the colonial format, they are yet not secure of their status and are in the upward swing marked A in figure 1.2.

If the other two cultures were much aware and skilled this part is now getting aware and skilled and is searching and identifying the need of their security and the status. This need could allow them to enter and reach the top of the third swing. A negative leader with his skills and awareness of the other two cultures may even try to prevent them to reach on the top but may in that case only be able to delay it. We would not discuss various possibilities that could come across independently if they have to follow. If the other two cultures start showing slightest fourth upward swing to it would automatically mean this culture is being taken care of their status and being given opportunity to come up.

The conclusion of the third decline

The region where western and the eastern culture exist today is of utmost importance for the entire mankind on earth. Summing up we would find that at the nuclei level at home and in family the love and affection is missing, as we go up in the society and the neighbourhood area the respect is not observed to be same. Further up in the sequence in the nation the leaders are on the place of pride who try to satisfy others ego. The other is a wide term which includes people of a wide spectrum of mental levels to be answered. The leaders clash here is not with the real achiever but with the persons in various fields who have some sort of leadership quality. Why is he trying to satisfy the ego of others? Because of selfish motive in him! The selfish motive is the biggest existing evil on earth today which has to be minimised and subsequently removed. Maintaining a positive approach in this concluding part we wish the western culture may continue to work in scientific development rapidly making the newer modes for improving the human standards and much more superior and advance. Simultaneously another section may again realise the importance of human values set by the virtue they have attained this height and think further to uplift the entire human mankind.

With globalisation and the fragmentation of people across the world the cultures described would no longer belong to any defined regional area. The dominance of each culture could be in the region they have come up but its penetration in other places would make the system heterogeneous. There would be people belonging of either of the cultural background in any part of the world. The churning taking place is to identify the new value of humanity in the recognised fashion which is accepted by a wide spectrum of people belonging to varying stage of their development of mind.

Let us wish that the eastern culture may try to fill the voids cropping in their existing pattern and may be able to make up the values stronger and may take the assistance from the former group in the field of living standards not to compete but to stay strong and healthy together. Let us wish these two together bring up the third culture which is quite below the standard.

The realisation of this uniform upliftment of human race ultimately would be the felt when the three cultures we have discussed ceased to exist and there remains a man for man or probably god for God.

Figure 1.1: more details,

In the curve we have following two parameters together,

1- First swing: Love and knowledge,

2- Second swing: Respect and awareness,

3- Third swing: Moral value and skills.

1- Love is one basic value that has to sustain through out and is the reason for movement forward. It is explained that love would mean basic need in an organisation; love would mean security in a national network. Thus in an expanded single unit the word of love could mean different but if the expanded unit is fulfilling the requirement of love it would mean that the individual is happy and returning the love to the society.

Knowledge word is associated here because it is the reason for the basic value and would remain always. The knowledge in an individual could be understood but same knowledge in inter human could create difference.

2- The respect as the second value is extrapolation of love when there are minimum two individuals, two groups, two organisation, two nations or any two units. Respect means trust and it there are two units involved together and have to move forward there has to be trust between them. The flow of trust between two would happen if there were no comparative statement such as superior – inferior, big – small. The boss would remain a boss irrespective of his showing by words of body language. If it is so the trust creates bond.

If the two units have to be together recurring interaction and understanding creates awareness, which has duality in nature. One can do good or even harm in awareness but where the trust is strong and both respect each other such thing should not happen. What we mean by a strong trust?

The communication flow from either unit is happening properly. Even if the subordinate is listening the order from the boss he is mentally free to suggest in return if he thinks there could be value addition. In this process each of them are open to listen others view and hence are open to acquire more knowledge. If we remember knowledge is the basic and they want to acquire more of it. The respect between such units could be said of commanding nature.

On the other hand if respect is of demanded nature that itself would mean the flow of knowledge is happening in one direction. If a boss demands the respect or the work the subordinate would follow and would not add any value. Even if boss is knowledgeable for the subject he is loosing the opportunity that his subordinate takes up his experience sooner to move further to add quality (in working, organisation or life). The knowledge gained by sharing and experiencing in addition or knowing more views for one thing are missed and so the progress does not happen or delay.

3- Similarly when there are more than 2 individuals (say 3 in numbers) respect itself falls short to work in cohesion. Moral value comes as we have read. If there are 3 close friends and they love each other, they respect each other the moral value has a part to play also. If at a time there are two of them present they would not discuss bad of the third not present. This is a simple law. All three trust each other such that their absence does not create another point of view among them. It is true for any different set of units when they are more than two. We have seen that nation is one format where it is required for good governance.

If the moral value were there it would again mean that there is a flow of knowledge among them. It would be easy to reach to a common action with clarity on the unknown aspect of the experiment, which could be corrected. It would also mean that each unit is agreeing to take responsibility and in such condition the growth would be in forward direction even there is a natural delay to avoid generation of wrong direction.

In fact it is the freedom of mind, which allows accumulating the knowledge, and filtering out what is not desirable. This could continue if in the largest unit when moral values are followed which would mean all units respect each other and further would mean there is love present in all of them.

More units do generate more problems and that we see in the world but in the process of metal evolution some one has to take a lead in a realised state to see entire world as one, with no disparity and create a reversible reaction from them. Time could not be ripe at present but that would be the next swing.

CHAPTER 2

THE LOGIC SENSE AND THE NATURE

Logic sense

We have seen that the development of the mankind has taken place in steps. It has passed through he tribal format and then in colonial form and then in national form. Though all the three formats still exist in raw form or in different developed form which has identical values to hold the unit, at each step they formed certain values and norms not by force but by the self, as it was the need of the time. Following those norms he was ale to *think* better and in the process he was able to define the path to achieve the internal pleasure which is a mental state of human being. It was again the man at every stage of the progress generated hindrance in trying to achieve a negative pleasure in stopping the growth. In the former case if was laying the path to lead to god in the later case he was trying to push even below the stage of animal kingdom from where he would have arisen and who have certain norms for survival keeping harmony with the nature.

The human like animal for survival had few essential requirements of food, a shelter and copulation to run the race. These basic requirements probably are sill unchanged. With the growth of the mankind the human behavioural pattern was changing at each stage, if he gained two things he lost one as well. From the very moment human developed a crack in the natural brain called as mind he had made big leap in a forward direction. If the ingredients of basic need and shelter or security spring from the unwarranted fear existing, he started thinking to confront the situation and find some way out by the natural resources. Gradually these resources which provided them to be sure of basic need led to provide them certain comfort. These comforts which were realised from the very beginning with time were re-defined as the development went on and explored in depth.

Let's discuss the origin of and bearing of these comforts which has a direct bearing with the values of the mankind. In the swinging mankind we have elaborated the swinging characteristics in terms of human values. In this journey the mankind has achieved three peaks so far. In each step of civilisation the man has been working to achieve the mental satisfaction in a higher degree and thus derive a pleasure from it. All along the growth of mankind a parallel activity was going on which relates to the physical comfort. It was the logic sense which was applied and continuously upgraded. Unlike the values and mankind, which saw peaks and troughs, the logic sense had only one direction to grow that is upwards. Around the peak of the sinusoidal curve there was a sharp evolution of results to change the habitat of the human. The increase of logics could be gradual because the strong roots were being prepared initially but as the end results the growth was exponentially at each succeeding peak they came across of tribal, colonial and national formats.

Logic sense and the changing need

The prime energy requirement comes from food and is the primary basic requirement. Let's start from this and from the point man became selective in eating habits. He started to eat food baked or cooked in heat which may be an accident to start with, he developed a sense of taste and never looked back to the raw stuff (flesh) which he was consuming earlier.

There would be exception existing on the day who eat raw fish but that does not stop from our basis of moving ahead in the evolution. With time it was not the matter of taste which bound them towards semi cooked and cooked food but his own body was not ready to accept the raw food. His stomach which receives the food for further processing in the changed condition of evolution became tuned to the refined food of the prevailing situation. If in the beginning he used to eat raw flesh, his stomach was ready to do the hard work to make other body organs function to the specific need at that time. With refined grade of food the workload had decreased and must have felt a sight of relief. After tuning to the new system if he consumed raw flesh again the stomach of evolved human was not ready to process leading to all sorts of pain and malfunctioning of the physical body. This made him to think for further refinement and not to go back.

The man was living initially in the natural state. They lived in nature with natural instinct and habitat keeping a natural balance. It was not only human but also the other existing nature such as animals and plantation including rivers; forest and climatic condition existed in balanced state. In the natural state the humans stayed naked, covering their bare body was the first act to lift them in the humanity level. This act of humanity also helped to cope with the vagaries of weather condition. In the process human body stated becoming weaker to resist the natural condition. If the body was felt becoming weaker it was the developing mind, which was opening to understand the difference. This difference in the mind that had cropped was non-returnable step since then and there has been only one-way to improve and improve.

In the process of the evolution with respect to human values we have observed the behaviour in sinusoidal curve where we have attained three peaks and three troughs. The rise of logic sense on the other side had a growth in only one direction upwards till the day. The extent of growth is exponential in nature at each peak they have achieved. The evolutionary process we have divided in three segments of tribal, colonial and national level. It was the successive peaks where such format was realised and adopted. It was the peak where the usage of the logics and consequently the through the inventions were used by more and more people. The peak therefore was the area that was generating satisfaction to the user of new knowledge. Stable and satisfied period also became the period for a rapid growth in specified regions where the state of evolution was ahead.

The fear of himself

It must have taken tens of thousands years initially for human to reach any significant value in terms of rise in logic sense. The reason is simple that in the earlier tribal era human pockets were scattered and there was no significant contact with one another. The human or other living species used to live near the natural water source for the supply of their basic need. Within this parameter evolved human of this era had started living in groups, more secured life now increased the life expectancy and thus increase of population. This more secured human was consuming nutritious meals, selective fruits and vegetables, selectively cooked meat and fish. As he did not eat grass and leaves he found cow, buffalo and goats that can live on them and provide them a ready made product as milk and flesh full of taste and value.

Selective vegetation habit and increasing population made necessity to produce crop and fruits and preserve them better. He was able to tame cow, buffalo and goat for milk. Gradually each separate group formed a habit for growing some crop and taming animals, which was their new method of living for their survival. It was the time when distribution of wealth was not in the knowledge and practiced.

They understood the art of farming, understanding the need of water for it though they were entirely dependent on the rain God. With the vagaries of nature and rain in excess or in deficit situation made them to think an alternative mode for the crop. Availability of water would not have been constrained as they were habituated near the water source. Development of wooden bowl for transfer of water must be the initial method towards it. There were no shortage of hands and thus the sharing of such responsibility for watering could have been satisfying in bonding them but the process was still cumbersome and not very effective. The brain power already had come in some refined form and if one section was busy in the fields there were other who kept thinking to improve the method for watering or defending the fields from the birds. With passage of time and changing food habits they realised farming as the most essential necessity related to the prime basic need and they were in no position to loose a crop because of lack of rain or any other natural calamity. This made them to think better ploughing and more efficient watering methods. If they relied on two hands they preferred more children for increasing the efficiency.

More people in a family or in a social group not only gave the advantage of assistance but also enhanced their moods and skills in work. In such a situation a sickness to any member was not to be easily left off. It probed the mind of some in the direction to find the remedy of the normal ailments that they suffered. If it was the fear of basic need which prompted them to develop skill in farming it was the fear of his life made him thought for finding the remedy of cuts, burn or disease which were prevalent at that time. They were able to identify certain piants or roots as a remedial measure for certain ailments and they must have derived a sense of success in that.

First effective step towards progress:

These improvements must have taken thousands and thousands of years and followed till a time we can assume them to be much improved human in terms of their habits of food, covering themselves and shelter. They must also have been connected with other tribal habitat or as to say their social group must have been expanded to a much wider area. With civilisation already coming in shape people aware of their basic need they were able to know more about different soil and their different crop bearing knowledge naturally in the existing atmospheric and climatic conditions. Invention of ploughing wooden instruments to assist was a remarkable achievement. If usage of such instrument was tiring he took the animal help to do the laborious part. The results were astonishing; their fatigue level was low with better output.

Realisation of Animal Power over the manpower was the first step towards the speedy progress in the logic sense. The maximum usage of animal power was the period which coincided with the first peak in the development of values. Once known the animal can contribute to increase the efficiency they saw different animals which can be tamed for different areas of need. Cows, buffalos and goats were for the milk and meat it was the ox for ploughing. Donkeys were found useful for carrying loads of materials on their back; horses were tamed to carry them to much farther areas. Human mind was definitely grown to a much higher order as where they were able to understand the brain and ability of animals now.

The other end of their growth was to understand their body. It is important to understand that in the civilisation at one step backward people did not have much of mental problem and worries and were not ambitious as well. Their problems were of lesser magnitude to that we can realise today but burns, cuts aches, muscle pull and stomach upset must have been there to bother. Temporary physical disorders because of their movement or food infection existed to be a concern. With hit and trial they were able to earmark plants, their extracts and natural resource such as milk, honey and ghee as a remedy.

The new dimension ahead

Period between the first decline and near the peak of the second peak (colonial era) the logic sense gradually progressed in steps which lead to the new dimensions in the scientific world. Once the man started using the animal power their access to the region were increased. They were able to commute and or carry material to the region far off. It could have helped in consolidating the religion or add the values existing other than what they knew. Gradually it could have led to exchange the ideas and even share the habitat. Barter system of exchanging material could have generated then in the preliminary stage could be for making friend without the actual word's meaning, which was followed after as a system. The dedicated group utilising their mental energy for the improvement had already taken man very far from nature. He was no more living in a mud hut only; he was no longer covering his body by plant leaves but by hand woven fabrics. He had found many basic metals to be useful as ornaments or as kitchen ware. The concept of increasing efficiency was realised with the invention of lever and its application at odd difficult places. It was the invention of gear and drive that brought the revolution.

With gear and levers in the beginning allowed them to change the motion and do harder job with lesser effort it was the invention of drive (motor) which changed the total scene of development. The utilisation of drive gradually was changing the meaning in every segment of their work, in farming, in commuting and as the base value in adding the logic sense.

The initial manpower was converted in steps to animal power, which was now being converted, into a machine power. The brainpower was now in the new heights and with the machine not only efficiencies were increasing but were able to do much difficult jobs which otherwise the man could never had thought of.

Another vital area of interest for the development was to understand the body. The need arose because of compulsion to prevent illness and reduce unnatural suffering. In the process to understand it, name was given for each of the organs and its role in the system and the generated the knowledge for basic input required for that organ. For example if any thing is eaten how it was accepted by the stomach which was the starting point for the processing of food. Further how the processing was carried out by various different organs to convert into the useful blood which is the life line. How the unacceptable part is rejected and secreted as waste through the kidneys and intestines. The role of the heart which caters the blood supply to the entire system was found out. With the knowledge of the system and its functioning the chemistry involved were found which lead them to understand of deficit or excess of certain chemicals in the case one is physically not well.

Human thought and found the method for the synthesis for such chemicals externally. They had to invent the ingredients to make the required chemicals, but nothing is impossible what a man can dream about. Now the question is, how it helped them? Any sickness was attributed because of decrease in efficiency of some part of the body causing imbalance and subsequently a state of dullness. With the knowledge of chemical that would have been short for the specified illness he extrapolated that in the state when a person is suffering from certain illness and is body is weaker and if deficit chemical is induced externally in the body the system could revive and bring back the body in the normal state. Such logic senses lead to the invention of alophatic drugs.

The total growth was being done on the reasoning and scientific logics. In the earlier time the cure was found in roots and extracts and the natural available substance called herbs but the effect was much slower. The slower process was not convinced to the scientist and thus developed such drugs. One of the simplest drugs made was aspirin, which till today is supposed to be effective.

Improvement in standard of living with the weakening of physical ability

We have to understand two facts very clearly in the chapter of development of logic sense which has the significance in over all effect in the movement of humanity till today.

1. The first peak of humanity coincided with the age of animal power which must have taken hundreds of thousands of years where as the second peak coincided with the mechanical power that must have taken another tens of thousands of years to reach. This is to tell that logic sense part played in the humanity growth is in linear in direction without any ups and down but each step forward or each milestone was nearer than the last one.
2. Understanding the development of logic sense which has also the bearing on the prevailing system. This is to say logics were not only the means for scientific advancement but each scientific development also in turn was utilised for the welfare in day-to-day activities to improve or reduce the values. It should be also understood that the development graph we would discuss would be of going upwards. That would not mean entire system or population was benefited form it but the one who is leading also would be the

pathfinder for others. This is similar as in the chapter of human values we discussed of the humanity rise leaving the sections which were or even today exist in different underdeveloped state. But positive moves have been the leading and the guiding factor.

Shaping of non agriculture area

In each step of development that the man was making he has been combating with newer problems of two types. One probably was not aware earlier and with the rise of logic sense he was becoming aware about it. The second one with development and changing behaviour pattern he was coming across newer types of problem unknown earlier. This did not stop him to look ahead. He took the challenge every time and met with a newer challenge ahead.

Let us discuss of the age between the decline of tribal era and the ascending of colonial era. The colonial format was essentially of much larger territory and governed by the leaders or a king. One colony comprised of different thinking and behaviour people and the leader or the king had to look for the welfare of all. Essentially he had to see that every one in his territory is able to get the basic need of food, cloth and shelter and has a feeling of security. With advancement of thinking definite social activities were formed which were the positive outcome by experience. Though the agriculture remained the main profession as the source of generation of basic need there was an emergence of non-agricultural activities. This section or part of this section had geared their logic sense and were responsible not only for adding skills for their counterparts in agriculture but to spread security, and promote social and cultural activities to educate the mass for the harmony and enjoying their life. The emergence of talents was there in the fields of art, music, architect and craftsmanship and areas of scientific knowledge. Accumulation of such talents was happening in a isolate place away from the farmland where they could promote their good cause in the state of tranquillity.

Generation of agriculture and non- agricultural section also necessitated the methodology to transfer the benefit of each to the other. These people did not snatch the food but a barter system thus was developed for fulfilment of the equation.

The development of non-agriculture sector happened in a separate place away from the farmland where the access of water was there and with availability of food grain distribution outlet. This immediately gave them the thought for change in life style. The houses were no more between the fields. They built spacious and simple apartments but with arrangement for sitting and relaxing. Change was there in the clothing and for a better look in these developed people. Need of proper road was there as movement was far more than their counter part in the fields. These non-agricultural activities of administration and guarding territorial security, spreading social and cultural development and other technical skills exhausted the people mentally more rather than physically as their counterpart in the fields were experiencing.

Pleasing achievement

Development in any section could be thought relating its application at home, work place or in between. People had started making houses of bricks, stones and with proper masonry work. As their leader looked after their daily bread it was their duty to make the leaders feel elevated and pleased. Big palatial bungalows were made with sturdier construction better in look and more comfortable in a natural weather condition. They were designed such that the houses were cooler in summer and warmer in winter. The houses for themselves though were built smaller but with similar concept of keeping open, well ventilated with lots of greenery around. In the process architectural skills were developed also generating physical work to satisfy another section.

On the social front if the leader was taking interest in spreading the knowledge across within his territory there were scholars and pandits who realised that how much the leader must be getting exhausted mentally doing the daily chores. To please him they invented humour, poems, songs and dances which were tension relieving doses. The art was enjoyed by all in palace and outside by the participants and the receiver be listening or and watching the shows. Such relaxation some time brilliant ideas to serve the people by focusing the prevailing issues in the forms of humour or poems in a lighthearted manner without touching the ego of the leader. Folk dances and songs were well existing in the past but the message and the melody was refined for mass appeal. Such social activity was spread in agricultural area also to mark a festivity mood for harvesting or any other occasion. This act was fruitful in maintaining harmony. Consequently the religion was nurtured in the community both in the developing agricultural and non-agricultural sectors.

The scientist had different thing in store who were equally concerned for the society. They were equally bothered for the mass and the rulers. Their effort and invention of pulleys levers and gears not only enabled to reduce the physical work but to do far more than they ever thought of. Generation of handloom sector for knitting the fabric emerged as a developing area as it related to one essential factor for covering themselves now in better shades. Discovering of newer elements and method for extraction of metals were the resource which gave new direction in time ahead. More and more people were employed to participate in these new ventures where people were working for the people. These hard working labour forces started working harder for more results and to get more return fulfilling their need and desire.

Semi urbanisation

With non-agricultural section already coming in shape a semi urbanisation was taking place. Demand of housing was increased and so for the work force to make it. Houses with a small garden kept the association with nature unlike palatial mansions full of natural surroundings for the leader or king. These houses gave a place to dwell and the security against the adverse condition of rain and storm like situations but the freshness in these houses were not the same as found earlier and a discomfort was there in a safe and secure dwellings.

Positive approach and the dedication had started showing good results for a large segment of population. Importance of arts and culture was increased and education was given priority in this section. New poets, new writers emerging, new rhythms, new dances and songs were developed, even musical instruments present were modified to give a better effect in the social front. The environment of autonomous where existed gave the people to utilise their mental skills in the scientific areas. With wheels already known and with existing natural waterfall scientist invented electrical power never to look back. In any electrical application its main feature is to make a drive to rotate or produce a resistance to generate heat. He was able to rotate a fan to make a room cool. He was able to generate the heat by the convector and warm the room. Now he was independent of sunrise or sunset for work or leisure with electrical power there to give the brightness even in the darkness of night. With electricity power coming in picture the mechanical age was being replaced fast by a rapid development of product useful in all the spheres of agricultural and non-agricultural sections.

With ultimate product being of public need at home or office or in the farm there was a large requirement generated for the production of products and thus chain of industries were set up for fulfilling the demand. Considering an example of a fan making industry of all metallic part it is made of metallic wings, screws and nut, a rod, motor and cover. The starting point was the metal extraction from the earth crust. Iron was extracted which was converted into ingots and other shapes for further use. The sheets, ingots, rods and of other shape material was then send to ancillaries for the fabrication of different components. Similarly another metal extracting company was responsible to extract copper from the raw earth crust. Copper was converted into wires which found the use in making a drive (motor). There were industries making nuts and bolts. One company was gathering different components and assembling to make the final product acceptable as the necessity of the day. Similarly each consumer item involved a string of industries to give final shape. In each case the electricity was the prime mover and with the increase in demand power generation became a full-fledged industry in itself. With industrialisation there was a requirement of work force and people from the farming started migrating in a non-agricultural set up thus formed. Urbanisation was taking place gradually which was seen as much developed area to that of agricultural part which still remained the source producing the prime basic need of people staying in farm or else.

With a non-agricultural sector becoming organised and work force increasing in abundance, requirement of land for dwelling was generated. In such situation residential locations were selected separately which were not by side of the water hole or river for the availability but the distribution network of water became necessary. The expansion of this region was associated with accessible roads for the fulfilment of their duties for their daily breads and also enabling them the interaction with the masses for the social commitments. The residential accommodations in the bulk were required but the sizes were getting smaller with the reduction of contact with the nature. In the changed condition of outer atmospheric condition, gadgets like the fan and cooler became a necessity. If one could not purchase them and living in the urban area they started aspiring for this materialistic thing born few decades earlier.

Development of urban and industrial sector was primarily done by the destruction of jungles and forests. The trees uprooted were used for carving the materials for offices and houses. Best wooden logs were finding the place for decoration of beds, tables and other furniture's for the comfort and pride of one section. Decorated pieces were carved to enhance the beauty of the house. If the best wood was the richest the next was for the second level. In the earlier time if the wood was used as a fuel the natural resource was maintained but now the greed of wood was being exploited.

Logic sense and the nature

We were going away from the nature in the changed environment which was self created. The nature is most superior which was not directly realised till this moment. If any part of nature was felt being lost the human was devising and developing a similar condition which in turn was made by the natural source. If the human was becoming or even feeling to be independent of nature in any department he had started becoming dependent on natural resources. If the nature is in abundance the natural resources are not, which was not the prime consideration. The reason that such development at the moment was limited in a small section of (so called) developed world and they had the knowledge and eye of abundance resource untapped in the rest of the world.

If the human had the pride to be independent of natural sunrise and sunset in his living and working did he not become dependent of electricity, fan, and pump sort of things? The human brain has never accepted defeat and at every stage he generated a new idea in practice. Necessity has been the mother of invention, truly and it would continue to be.

The logic sense was the core for all the development that had taken place. The interpretation of basic logic was made and various hypotheses were made which were verified by various experiments. In such process human mind was able to invent, which as a end result gave ease in their part of their work and or gave additional comfort in living. The user of the other part started using all the developed facilities for the sake of their pride that they can possess and may have created a sense of comparison to the one who actually needed and were not able to afford. People belonging of both the groups would never think that some one due to his hard work and devotion did such invention. Such person belonging to the former group never utilised the devised facility. The creative mind and dedication yielded the results and was the cause for him to derive the pleasure. He not only invented for the betterment of the growth but also gave the direction to a person like him to develop further in modifying the invention or giving an idea in his creation from the root as basic.

The development in engineering and medical fields were in spate and in the machine age. He had developed enough knowledge about his body and functions and much more in the mechanism and the reaction occurring in the body. He was able to draw a clear analogy between the industry and the human body which was like a full-fledged industry which carried out all the possible operations of engineering with a flawless technique. It was the ideal machine which he has yet to produce. He is yet to find out how it converts and extracts in such a exact proportion to keep the body mechanism perfect. If even one of the known composition he has to prepare synthetically he has to use dangerous / poisonous chemicals, has to keep manufacturing condition of high and low pressure and or temperatures where as the body in the absence of any such condition does the job perfectly.

Urban living

Up till now we have discussed the primary development needed in the process of urbanisation. The end application related to the comfort at home or at working place of the people. As the positive doers were shaping the civilisation up gradation in one section of the world by following a path of values with certain norms such people were also aware of the changed living situation that was developing. The major area that the leader had to look was the basic need of the people, spreading the social culture and maintaining the security but in the changed situation. The transportation and communication required the face-lift as a necessity to keep the continuity of the development. Let us go through the sequence of development on few of such areas which still remain important for making the benefit reached to the masses as the ultimate goal.

Transportation

Importance of the transportation was realised since ages. Donkeys and camels were used to transport material and human in comparatively short distances. Horses were used in wars in the earlier era. Towards the age of mechanisation it was not only individuals who were to be transported but more important was it required to transport the food stock for the distribution from agricultural to non agricultural area. Food being the prime concern for distribution but with industriali-sation entire network was dependent on the transportation. It was the lever and wheel concept, which gave the bicycle concept a self-driven vehicle. It required the art for balancing and made man bit independent of animal for going few kilometres and had the limitation of person and material transfer which was their goal. Scientist realised the strength of the steam and coal based locomotives were developed. This was the first step towards the growth in transportation useful to a larger society gradually the rails were spread and its potential to carry load was understood. Transportation seemed easier to a long distance with minimum physical effort. The movement was restricted to the areas where the rails where laid down. There was also the requirement of linking two urban areas. Invention of small diesel engine and subsequently a motorcar filled this gap. A car was comparatively a small vehicle which was capable to move in much inaccessible region. With urbanisation spreading the utility of this car became very important.

For the individuals the basic need remain the same of food, clothes, shelter and security and if administration was a vital requirement in such situation the transportation became a full-fledged sector to fulfil the job. Motorcar at this point was a gift to the people and made them independent of worries of distance this comfort in movement added a linear growth in their ability. Trade being the prime mover in the growth of a nation only inland movement was not sufficient and the man thought to enter the other world across the sea.

Boats were used in the river since a long time. By now the man built big ships which could move in the wild tides of the sea. The diesel engine invention was used in this area as well when he was ale to make massive ships. Transporting huge load of material across the sea was now equally easy.

Touching the area across the sea was an achievement in much larger sense. The process facilitated exchange of materials but more importantly gave the opportunity to come in contact with another world within our world with absolutely different customs and habits of the people. Sharing and exchanging the views with the different lot of people gave a scope for the growth. Inland or across the sea the transportation was vital to control the civil administration at the national level and for the industries which had become an integral part of the development of society and the growth of the mankind.

Communication

There was another important sector shaping gradually to meet the demand of the growth. Gone are the days when the king had almighty human force with a fleet of horses and messenger were there to convey the message across their territory or the appointed ministers conveyed the message by going round the town with beating drums to call attention of the people. Those were the time when the message flow was important to flow in one direction or as thought to be by the leaders. Communication in one direction can lead or perish but would lack the development part which is essential. No development means stagnation means death.

In the era where certain industrialisation had taken place, certain social development was set and re-set communication gave a code of conduct in the behaviour pattern of people. It had become important to convey and receive the messages. Letter was one method to the transfer the message but in the mechanical age of advancement faster modes were required. Telephone was invented where two persons connected through a cable were able to communicate by talking and hearing. This invention also helped in the invention of teleprinter to communicate in writing where by certain symbol codes the message was transmitted to a known party on the other end of communication situated far away. Socially it was great achievement and controlling became simple.

Now a person sitting a home was able to know what is happening in his industry. He was confident for achieving the desired goal by faster information be it for fulfilling to market his product or getting the raw material or even for giving guidance to one of his pupil.

Comfort and the mistaken pleasure

Transportation and communication were two great achievements and became a primary need in the developed society for controlling the policies within the boundaries of the nation and for controlling the industrialised sector. If the motor car and telephone gave comfort, gradually they became a necessity to one section. Such gadgets were also associated with different social implication. Communication with a dear one situated at a far off place was also possible and that made many others to aspire for it.

Outcome of these innovations realised as facilities were in the great help of those who were putting hard work for their goals in any field and such people were motivated in promotion of their growth and consequently the growth of the social and the nation.

These facilities formed an integral part of their life and also added pleasure in it. Pleasure is the ultimate which every one would like to attain (though definition of pleasure also would change with time and understanding) and if gadgets like motorcar and telephone would give the pleasure every one thought to possess them. In fact it was for only the hard working people that such gadgets facilitated in their promotion of their work. In such a situation it was the hard labour and the devotion, which gave the pleasure not the gadgets, but on the other hand those people who did not know this were also not ready to know with their sole aim to acquire such materials. Such people were intending to spoil the ethics and the culture and even if they were successful in acquiring they did not derive the pleasure and were far from snatching the pleasure from the devoted people who actually were enjoying it. There started an unsaid war of ethical and unethical practices.

Was a person not becoming weaker mentally on this area?

Mental strings to metal strings

Every step of such development was contributing to make human independent of natural situation when he was able to work for more hours in a day. The darkness of the night was no longer a barrier, the car made to reach unimaginable distances in a shorter time and communication with another far of did not bother him. Such habits were converting his mental sphere blocked with all sorts of tangible and intangible thoughts, as many were not ready for change. If he was able overcome physical labour by utilising the inventions now he was feeling much more mentally tiring.

In the rapid development era of mechanical age there was one section realising the burden of the mind which the people were facing and they had to offer something to calm down the turbulence of mental strings. Birth of great laureates, writers and poets were there, songs and dances were being promoted. The literature and poetry were made to read and listen by the people, which helped in knowing the experience and or the way of highlighting the weakness of a system or of the leader in a lighter spirit. It helped to educate oneself keeping his ego one side if that was the cause for his mental block knowingly or unknowingly.

On the other hand the songs and the dances had the rhythm which attracted the eyes and the mind of a mentally busy person and gave them a break in part of their thinking process which resulted to give them a satisfying pleasure. The ability of these arts were not attached with material were directly related to the art of self of human. It had the strength to regenerate the strain of mental exhaustion. The art was later on developed with various instruments and rhythm developed appealing to the people. Songs and dances existed ever since the social groups were formed in their customary fashion. Folk songs and dances were known since the ages as an occasion for celebration to share and show happiness. The importance can be compared of the developed mechanical age to that of tribal era when such occasion gave them the opportunity to strengthen the bond of love in the community and gave the added pleasure in their life. In the changed and developed situation even the hard working section that were busy in fulfilling the goals for a nation were finding less time for human interaction apart of the work. Unknowingly he was loosening the bond of love with humans and in such a situation, music or song or dance or poetry gave him an opportunity to get away from his mental strings, relax and derive an overall feeling of enjoyment.

These arts were acting as regeneration strength to the mind of the people. To overcome the debacle of the mental pressure being faced by the hectic activities the songs, dances gave them the sense of aloofness from the connected worries and resulted in soothing the body and the mind. It was the art of the human body be his /her hands, legs or throat which were responsible to switch over his worries. No doubt it was human art which was and would remain superior to the material in the world.

It was not only in the state of worry that the music or dance was rejoiced. A happy and healthy person enjoyed and infact he was in a much superior state to appreciate or participate. The importance of the art and the skill therefore was realised in every aspect. Being so important the development of each part be dance or a vocal recital or an instrument playing or combination of them had a place for their growth and promotion.

Capturing the sound

The importance of the art would never have been realised unless it was spread in the masses. The invention of gramophone and radio were for filling the gap where the skill was straight brought in contact wit the people living in the most remote area. The invention was not only for the entertainment but it was possible to pass on the information to the general public or masses.

Being the source of entertainment and the masses need the broadcasting methods and systems were improved even the gadgets saw gradual improvement from a large size radio with ability to catch few stations to smaller in size with better receiving abilities. It became a necessity with time rather than the source of luxury and was developed to suit the pocket of masses.

The invention of a radio was a remarkable achievement which normally one would not even think today. The conversion of sound energy to electrical and back to its original was by no means a small task. He had discovered the characteristic and behaviour pattern of sound waves and mode of is movement. If the sound waves were transmitted trough cables initially micro wave link were established with years to follow and on the day any distance of the world is no barrier. It has become one of the most powerful media to connect people of any part of the world.

The invention of sound and its transfer method and the knowledge of the strength in communication people developed the method the capture the sound on a disc. If the great artist or leaders was supposed to have high capability in the subject capturing their sound was a guiding factor to many through the indirect means. It has certainly helped the world in the growth towards a speedy development and the surface more hidden talent in the process.

Transformation age with weakening of ability

The logic application in the human started right from the moment their eating taste was shifted from the jungle law which could be of tasting of cooked or baked flesh. The developing mind worked in the areas of their basic requirements of food, shelter and security. Gradual farming was one of their main professions. The development passed through the region of animal power and in step reached the mechanical age. From this point rapid development in science caused the upsurge of industrialisation. Farming having its role to play using the technology, industrialisation generated urbanisation which was catering a big role in social and security of the nations.

With growing need for a speedy development and climatic condition in their favour to work there was ushers of invention cropping up as we have discussed like in the field of transportation, communication and many more. The new modes and the media developed did help various segments of social, cultural, and administrative level of civil work and thus a different cultural heritage was mushrooming in the urban area. Food may have been still the prime requirement but farming activity was not in the priority for the people staying in the urban area. The majority of the people in the urban area working in the social sector, education sector civil administration or industries were following a defined job. These people were assigned some specific routine work and in return they did not have the power to think of real pleasure of mind, their approach narrowed down to have all the facilities (material) which they thought their leading personalities were using to fulfil their herculean task. Where as these materials were the source for doing extra work and extra effort for fulfilment of their mission for the social benefit the majority of the followers thought saw it as the added luxury and aspired to achieve it without their share of dedication on the work.

The advancement of logic sense the ultimate benefit of the product be of engineering or medical or other nature was directly either as a luxury or a device to improve the efficiency in the work. Scientist may have invented for a common goal of the humanity but the beneficiaries were lesser and lesser in each step of advancement. This is represented in the figure IV below,

Figure-2.1

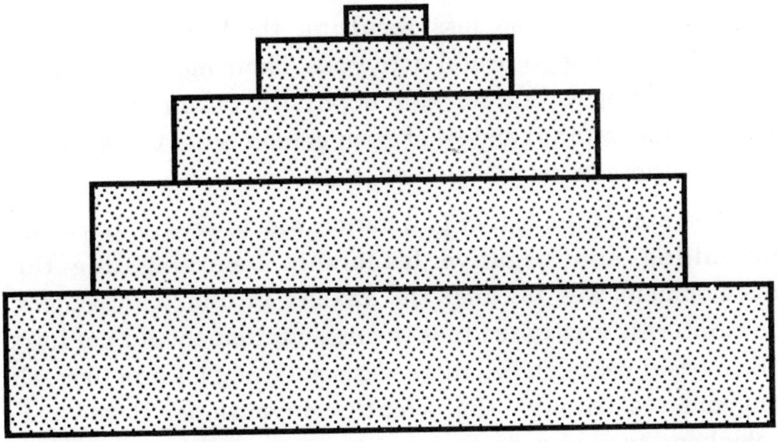

Advantage of development in the decreasing population

With so much of development in the mechanical age invention of electricity had brought the transition age with much rapid growth. If the scientific innovation were made for the human growth they were not thought for any specific segment particular but what was happening in actual was not the same. With each step of development there was step being formed as in the figure IV. Facilities like transportation, communication were invented to facilitate the growth of mankind and persons essential to posses were the dedicated ones who served the masses. These were the positive people who were utilising the extra mental activity for the welfare of the humanity at the cost of lesser physical labour. These were the dedicator nation movers, industrialist and the social workers.

So much said about the positive people and using the comfort but primary development was utilised by majority section in farming or industries or other social groups. The people who were doing their job to earn their bread and butter also were experiencing much lesser physical labour. Among such people if they lacked the spirit at times the mental exhaustion was also less resulting their mind to think elsewhere in not so useful activities. Their mental faculties were becoming weaker for want of physical labour (which they did not understand) and what such person could think was to exploit others in his group or co-group.

The aim of the leader of a nation was to see the harmony prevailing and negative leadership emerging due the development was to cause the anxiety in him. The leaders' first interest was to see that the exploitation should not hurt the masses peace and so there was something for him to reach the masses through the scientific inventions. If the car, telephone type of gadgets were creating a self in a section of people the other side there the audio transmission was found to be one of the powerful media to reach the masses by the leader. Broadcasting and relaying being one major form for transferring the message was utilised by them to control the sentiments and it was kept under the control of the governing body.

Controlling may be done to restrict the exploitation but the fact it was controlled itself would mean the message to be biased in nature. In absence of healthy criticism the growth towards a positive development is restricted

Controlled by a single body would mean the orientation would be from the point of view of that functioning body unchallenged which itself would mean under utilising the potential available. Within a nation it could have helped (or may be helping) the national leader to maintain an ideology but humanity does not have any boundary. Radio transmission was also responsible to make aware the people what was all going in the other nations. After any amount of knowledge the total awareness is the correct step by which some one can add the value where as such advancement were also generating the half knowledge and a dangerous one for the society.

The upright leap

We have reached a threshold point of development where logic sense had made human reach to the new heights. In the graph of sinusoidal curve of the chapter-1 probably the growth has reached the distance near the third peak. The population of urban areas were increasing very rapidly and every one to live here required the support of the basic need. If the food distribution outlet were made within a short span and the easy reach water was equally important ingredient. The architects were in the limelight to plan for the living. The progress of housing sector now instead spreading horizontally the accommodation started becoming smaller and moved in the vertical direction. Two floors, four floors and it crossed many more floors. In moving upward whatever small gardens people were having was not considered to be important. In such small area the population became manifold and added movement burden on the road. Road, passage and the transportation systems were modified to cater the new generated need. This was the era when urban people had least contact with the nature.

We thought we have become independent of nature.

But is it true?

Maybe it is the prime question to bother the world. We have become dependent on natural resources in the process of every day as a part of our living.

The story of next step starts here to answer what logic sense had further in store as the process has to find newer method and redefine the changing situation and the requirement.

Electrical power was the basic energy for the growth and was required in every part of the life. Its demand was growing and different methods were devised to generate it. Utilising the rivers and natural falls, hydroelectric power was generated. As it was not sufficient coal was used for increasing the demand but this resource also had the limitation of quantity and the quality. Knowing that he is totally dependent today at least human is bothered for tomorrow and makes the effort to find an alternative source that would not exhaust. Human developed nuclear energy, which was a super achievement. Small amount of resource was required to generate very large amount of energy. It was supposed to be the resource of tomorrow but sooner he realised this source as more powerful than himself, a small error could lead to human catastrophe.

The entire development can be visualised by our own body and system. The pumps are simulated from the function of the entire digestion, functions were simulated in industrial application to convert natural source to the useful matter. The machines were replacing the job of hands and the mobility of legs were brought in motor driven system. He could not tolerate the freedom of birds in the sky and so had developed aircraft to fly.

At this step of the development, the contribution of poet and writers were very important for the up-liftment of the growing society. In this level of advancement if the writers and poets made all sorts of imagination and fiction to provide pleasure to the people, on the other hand the scientists were bent upon converting those fictions into realities. The basic purpose was to orient the development either to facilitate better living by substituting the smallest manual work by the machine or to speed up the job.

Jet age or the nose dive

Development had speeded the life of at least one section of the world community and had reached the jet age or electronic era. The existing car, buses and trains were improved to run faster the aeroplanes were made of gigantic size to cover larger distances and in a shorter time. When it was simpler to reach the other part of he globe crossing all the natural barriers of mountains, forest and oceans he was able to interact with more people of the world and exchange the development skills with them. Communication by phones and radio through the cable link was not possible and thus knowledge of sound was correlated with the object moving above the earth and transmitting the sound in the other direction. Satellites were made to cut the barriers in communication. This invention also found the increased activity for expanding the commerce and trade between the countries.

What artist has to contribute to the scientist?

Artist is one who tries to bring a man closer to reality or to take away from the turbulence he is surrounded by. If the paintings we draw are close to the actual, the eyes have a soothing effect on seeing it. Camera was also developed earlier, which also gave the opportunity to capture the images. As we were going away from the natural living and loosing the nature the photograph helped to make aware and find out more about the beauty of the nature.

The art of photography and invention of satellite enabled

the man to watch down the earth, so as what is in the store as viewed from a quite distance above the earth. This art was utilised for the information for identifying the air current over the earth and a possibility to foresee a tycoon or sever tidal waves shaping up somewhere in the sea. Such climatic prediction helped in warning the people of the region that could be affected.

There was another side of such development when people started using such technology for spying in the other country, which was negative in character. The invention of aeroplane, rockets and nuclear energy had already taken place. Knowledge of these hi-tech machines had other dimensions which were evolved by the negative mind as destructive machines. Since the natural state of living there was a territorial urge which is even in animals for their survival but that instinct was with keeping in nature in harmony. The same territorial instinct had come out in developing the weapons and destructive nuclear device in the name of safeguarding the territory of a nation. It was an inhumane development made to satisfy his ego of superiority over others, never the less it was there in the mind.

In the jet age when a person is becoming more lethargic physically and improving the mental skills the growth further can be subdivided mainly in three directions namely,

1) For his comforts,
2) Know more about himself and
3) Unimaginable exploration of the world.

1) For his comforts

The logic sense would grow linearly. First and foremost in developing any thing that would give him comfort. The definition of comfort though changes with time his approach has been to modify with the latest science in shaping them. If the machines had reduced the manual labour he was still not satisfied with the little amount of work he had to do on the machine. His reliability with the machine was so much in terms of quality that if machine was fed or told to do any operation it would preciously do where as man was expected to make an error.

Automation of process and of any part of operation was done. The machines were made to do specific operations on the signals of button. It improved the quality and the productivity and was appreciated by the user industries.

How ironical situation has become? The same man or the perfect animal was now having more faith on the machine. If we in the course of development went for industrialisation to give the fruits to a common man and spread the civilisation beyond the limit, those working force itself became a burden and automation became effective tool to minimise the human part and the industrialised population. This is still a matter of concern today in the world. We have to find the alternative avenues for the displaced force of the world or else we may see the clash with the developing mankind.

Let's see another area which was developed and had enormous social impact. We have said about the development of photography. Capturing the picture in a photograph was to confirm 'seeing is believing'. This art was extended in cinema, which became a source of entertainment for the people. The audiovisual cinema had a big hand to play in social awareness but it was still available for the urban area.

Knowing the strength of this medium scientist had in store the invention of audiovisual media of television. This invention had an added dimension in coming in contact with the masses. As in the case of audio system of broadcasting this media was to be controlled by the governing body of the nation to give information in the good taste of the country.

With audiovisual aid it was possible to give actual effect on mind. It was lacking to give the sense of feeling and taste but was capable to alter the mental orientation and generate sentiment like feelings.

Is it not the story that our grandfather told us which scientist turned into reality, push the button and you can watch what was happening around the world? Today it is the most powerful media which can influence for good or bad in the existing social scenario. People are happy seeing the world sitting in their home, which otherwise they would never have dreamt about.

Perhaps in the process of being aware about the world we are getting unaware about ourselves and the result is that we see a sharp drop in the social activity.

2) Know more about himself

In the electronic age and in the process of further refinement at each step we are putting mankind at stake. He is bound to be a troubled person. If physical ailments are less at work we have newer problems towards the mental side which is increasing more all the time. On the physical side also unnatural damages are rising because of the man made problems. To meet this challenge the medical science is equally developed towards the jet age.

He has found the technique to operate and rectify upon most of the vital organs. A lost eyesight can be regained, hearing problem can be overcome by a device. Damage in heart, kidney, intestine can be operated simply as the machine is overhauled. He has attempted to reach inside the body and correct or even change the organs and give a new life to the patients. As a step ahead some life saving risky operations are converted into much easier one such as balloon surgery for the heart blockage. With development in science and medicine the technique are also made sophisticated to work with great precision which is essential to assist doctor in their task.

Today it is possible through scientific advancement to fertilise an egg outside a mothers womb. He has found the basic DNA structure, which in the human cell is said to hold the key to a persons characteristic. Probably this could lead to alter the structure of the basic molecule to remove certain deficiencies to make a perfect baby which could possess all the qualities that his parents want him to possess.

With newer invention in the field of medicines they must be even working upon the one to make him immortal. It might sound like a fairy tale but who knows the medical science reaches that state as well. Probably the medical engineers are experimenting with the highest natures' gift known as human. He knows that the human is the perfect and ideal machine and wants to duplicate it. If this happens the consequences are unimaginable but let it be a fiction till that moment.

But do we know what is happening in the present time? There remains something still to call the nature great. The man is able to make a break through in the preparation of a medicine for a newly known disease. Just when he thinks he has overcome the problem there is another unknown fault detected in the best nature's machine (body) and it keeps on happening continuously. The mind fails to understand in this area. It does not know how the body would react to a new changed situation, which a person is attaining in his process of evolution. On one side attending a heart blockage has been made very simple the other side there are cancer ailments where he does not have enough clues for the cure. In the mad race the man has also come across a new virus by the name AIDS which is deadly enough to finish a large chunk of population in a short time. There could also be a probability of such a virus unknown till then could cause a havoc in the mankind without giving enough time to the genius for finding the remedy.

It is not only the medicine but the man has developed unmatched tools in aid of various cures. Instruments have been developed which can exactly inform and show the internal part of the body that has the defect. The machines are able to diagnose the sex of a newborn in the womb that is no longer mystery. He can still not have a choice of sex for the newborn and if he invents such a thing it would again hit back to the existence and thus the mankind.

The medical science development is carried out for the health and good cause of human being each development have some side effects touching the human values for which the man stands high. In the electronic or the jet age the medical science is putting the values of mankind at stake. If the man is not going to die where would the population stay and if he does not follow the need to copulate then what is he going to do ? The aim of the life would change and probably it would be even difficult to make a fair tale of such a time.

3) Unimaginable world exploration

Ever since the logic has turned scientific people have made theories and tried to prove their hypothesis by various calculations and ultimately which led to develop some sort of utility tool to the mankind. The human brain understands the logic and he manipulates the system. Here we reach the third sub section in the context for the development of unimaginable exploration. The machines and the automations, which were the substitutes of hands and the legs in all the sectors including farming, had improved quality and the quantity of life. Now the man saw his mind more loaded and thus thought to reduce its burden. Set calculations were fed in calculators, which gave them the results promptly with accuracy. With time ahead computers were invented to calculate theories and calculations. Basic science and the mathematics were utilised in the machine to follow a set rule as per the instruction and generate a prompt output. The function of a computer is based on the logic fed and when the question is fed in accordance to the code or language the machine generates the results of his interest. If the human has been great animal it was because he had a brain and the logic sense. If the man developed his logic sense for allround development now he has made a machine (computer) which has a logic sense too but with a variance. The machine can operate with buttons and limited to the logic it is fed. Probably the scientist is planning to develop a machine with a logic sense and would be able to do the job of a man.

Is it not the irony? The man is thinking to make a machine more intelligent than himself and if he does so it is difficult to predict the outcome and such success could lead to what consequence is still far to imagine.

The last fear

The logic sense, which was the starting step of evolution of mankind, has reached a situation where he has the last fear for his existence. This is the cross road to a big challenge ahead. If we divide the growth of science in medical and engineering we find that in the medical science a human in the process of finding a cure to any ailments and ability to alter or change the body parts are trying to make man a machine where as the engineering science are developing higher end computers with an aim to make the machine equivalent or more than a man.

Both the cases are against the nature and the natural state. It is also the fact that the man would be losing something (may be unknown) by moving far away from the natural state. Such a development might end up with an unpredictable end of mankind itself. It may lead to unnatural calamity which he may not know at present but the law of nature would follow to bring back the stable natural state.

This is not any special vision but the scientists themselves foresee with a fair amount of accuracy and have taken as a big challenge not to be defeated. In the jet and electronic age with a good knowledge of navigation and aeronautical expertise the scientist are exploring the world which has not been the existing place at the present. Humans have reached Antarctica for this reason. They are impressed by the purity and the clarity of the nature and are able to see the potential of the place. Presently the climatic condition being unfavourable the research might be to find the material resources but if any unnatural circumstances can be created by mankind, the place could be heaven for some if not all. The territorial fight has been a natural habit for any species existing including the humans safeguarding their national boundaries. In the case of Antarctica exploration many countries have reached there but in the depth of them with a same fear of mankind and only if they do not divide this area it would be a success as exploration for a common goal for the good of the human. Such a situation may never come as well nevertheless it has given an opportunity at least to a human to think of mankind beyond the limits of nation a reason to be happy for the survival of the human race.

The saving instinct of the human race does not limit to the earth but scientists have opened the avenues for exploration beyond the earth in the vast universe. Scientist are sending space shuttle near the vicinity of other planets to find out the atmospheric condition and to find out if life exist or the probability if life can exist there. Scientist are experimenting to identify the methods to travel in absolute different conditions of atmosphere and gravity to overcome the long journey if made to the planets. If the primary basic requirement is the food they are finding technique to grow the crops in a synthetic atmosphere to feed them in the tiring endless journey to the other part of the universe.

With sufficient knowledge of the atmospheric condition and ground composition of some of the planets scientist have found that the situation is adverse for the (human) existence at least in the few planets, which are nearer comparatively. The scientists are studying to find a technique for plantation that can be grown to change the ecology by simulating a similar condition as known to be there in the planets in the laboratory. The fear of survival has forced the scientist in the Herculean task in the exploration of universe. In fact the human have already achieved the first distinction by sending three astronauts on the moon. It would be not wrong to say that the three persons who went to the moon have done the most remarkable job in our human history till date and the two who have stepped on the moon surface are the greatest hero we have had on earth to guide others with time to come.

All along the path of evolution the great brains, devoted and dedicated scientists have kept on looking for the solutions and paved a path for a better living. Now it is the turn of each human on the earth to contribute and assist for the survival of our own human species. One day it may be possible to transfer human to another planet, it could be possible that they change the ecology of the planet to suit us and give a new dimension. Let us wish success to such an achievement, a unique milestone in the human life to keep the human superiority on top for which every man will have to shed his ego problem against the nature and the natural state and avoid becoming a synthetic animal dependent on every type of artificial resources.

CHAPTER 3

THE HUMANITY ELEMENT

The Humanity Element

In the first chapter we discussed about the evolution of the mankind. We have further seen how the values were able to create stability in the existing system. With time those values were not enough and prompted certain anti-value, creating instability. The stability was restoring again when the system was replaced by advanced new value. Thus we saw a pattern of mankind evolution, which was in sinusoidal nature with three troughs (high points) and three crests (low points). The high and low point represents a definite period with the changed style of the human.

The evolution has been mainly of the mind and the change therefore related to the changed meaning of the similar subject in the different type of set as he was passing through. We have used terms as "love", "respect", "moral value" and "humanity" and said to be the core values existing. These values would guide us through the cycle but it requires a proper interpretation.

In the tribe formation the love was the first value which was discovered responsible for keeping the stability in a small flock of people together. In such a time it was only love the essential element, the other values such as respect, moral value and humanity were all imbedded within them. Within that small group the love value allowed them make all the laws which was liked by all which automatically took care of other higher values generated later on. Therefore we see the higher values were generated with the changed pattern of the living community. In the changed pattern the units were increased and so the interrelation was becoming complex. To answer the relation of complexity we used the core values which are enough to give stable situation if understood properly.

In the world today we have probably all the forms and stage of evolution existing and thus the requirement of them differ and cannot be the same. There are still unprobed areas where the civilisation has not started and human are very near to the tribal era that must have been. Kingdom rule still prevails in many places which appear to give a national type of frame but they are still governed by a leader or a king. Accordingly different parts of the world are in different format, some are on the higher level of evolution where as the other still lack in the progress and thus there cannot be a direct compatible to each other but require different ingredients for their fulfilment.

There is another angle which is of our interest and understanding. Every individual whether he belongs to any place and any format in the world has a small world around him or her and not necessarily has to know much more. Every such individual also is governed by the same law of values and thus is important to interpret them.

One person is a unit, a family, a joint family; society, town, state, nation and the world can be the biggest unit. Each part of such unit plays an important role in the total larger format. Other important units developed in the process of development are industrial organisation, urban society could be for administrative or education or any other existing place where people add their contribution to the society and make their living. So is in the agricultural sector. Let us take one unit as one industry. A small workshop could be one of the smallest type of industry. It would mean it is driven by one person and few working towards the growth and such unit would resemble a tribe and their values would be relevant. To grow stronger the value is love and which would mean a relation compatible between the owner and the worker. Even if the worker do not get best package and they may not be having many clauses in contract there is unsaid and unwritten contract which bind them. The workers are ready to work 24 hrs if required and the owner takes certain requirement of those individual for them to feel comfort. If such situation is present the workshop is bound to grow. The industry could be bigger in size where there are necessarily many departments and where certain norms are required to pass the message form one point to the other. Or in other terms such industry has few departments, each department could be itself like a workshop in the requirement where the value important is love where as in the larger sense in that organisation the respect value is important to bind between the departments. Similarly a very large organisation having many branches in the country or in the world requires moral values. Coming back to the workshop level the value for stability is love. What does here love mean? Love here is the understanding between the owner and the worker by which the worker is able to fulfill his minimum family requirement and personal need. Between the owner and the worker, respect and moral values do not surface out but they are strongly embedded within love. Same organisation if grows to the next level where respect comes in existence the few people who where involved in love-bond stage occupy the place of authority because the respect was already there which has now surfaced out and could be the best form to link between the owner and the down working level. An industry could be straight away in the region where the respect value is important. So in a different unit set up the same core values play part responsible for individual or the larger unit as an individual which could even be a nation.

The second chapter we discussed is about the logic sense. The development was due to the human mind and the mind works on certain logics which are independent of values. The growth in science, engineering and medical and every part of the human activity today are for that reason. What is important to know that improvement in logic has reduced the manual / physical work but has increased the mental work. Man has become weaker physically and to compensate, it started utilising the comfort and in due course where he is losing the grip on bountiful nature but at the same time he is becoming dependent on natural resources. Dependence on natural resources is a definite cause of worry as the natural resource is limited. It should be understood that a big civilised section today may not be using all these resources but they are not directly our concern, as if any damage is expected or some reformation is required, it is the top priority.

The values and the logic are two variables which work together in any individual or any unit existing. There inter relation is complex and the best it could be understood by the theory of element.

The elemental theory

Humans and God :

Before the logic sense had struck the superior animal this species was existing as other animals and behaving in their own way for survival as seen in the jungle today. We are not interested in the jungle rule but GOD had created this creature for one of his greatest experiment conducted on earth. It could be to know if any creature on earth can understand HIM. To commence further he chose this super animal for experiment and gave him the logic sense. From that very day the they became the superior species, called themselves humans and consequently formed a community and then onwards he has been marching forward through different types of tribal, colonial and the national format. He is still marching forward and the stage has come when GOD calmly sitting in the heaven awaits the results of this creation. The situation on earth is different where the human community is trying to compete with HIM.

The element essentially consists of nuclei attached in the core. It has molecules and atoms which orbit around the nuclei. Molecular can be said to move in the outer orbit where as the atoms move in the inner orbit. We would be analysing the human values on these ground and then observe the similarity which exist.

Growth of the nuclei of mankind

Interpolating the mankind hypothesis we have fund that after the logic struck the first great value achieved was LOVE. Love was the bonding force which led to the emergence of tribes. The love bond was the first significant factor which was away from the natural instinct. If sex is also love, mother caring her child is also a love which is present in all living being but now this love had a variation attached with a mental state that made him feel more secure. Initial tribal people did not have the intelligence to think for pleasure and satisfaction. When they lived in small pockets together they copulated and nurtured a family. The feeling of security and the safety was brought in the picture for the survival of their species in the changed situation of additional knowledge. Thus the nuclei of the mankind was born where a self and his family together formed the core of the nuclei which is represented as B in figure 3.1

Figure 3.1

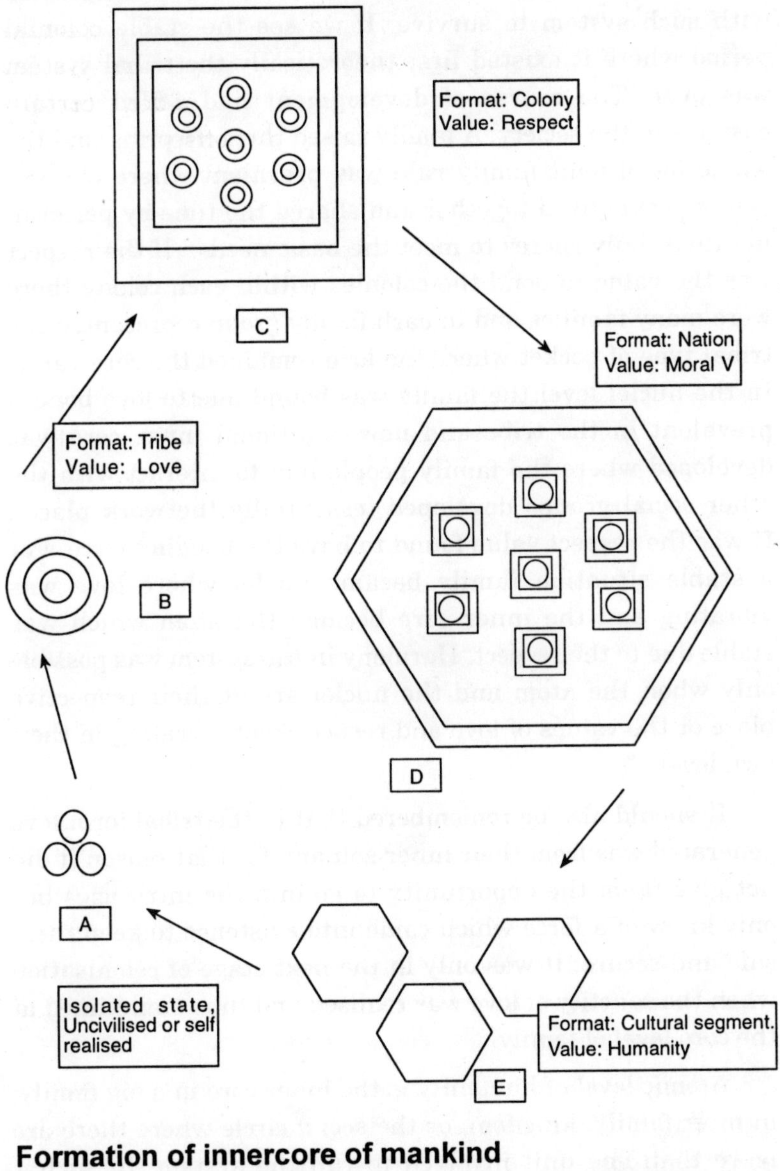

Formation of innercore of mankind

Moving further in their path of evolution small pockets of tribe came together and formed a colony with different values and systems. Respect was found to be the value associated with such system to survive. If we see the stable colonial period where it existed first theoretically the tribal system was over. The course of development had added certain customs in the society. A family raised their offspring and the whole lot of joint family rule was prevalent where old and young people lived together and shared the time by performing their daily chores to meet the basic needs. If the respect was the value to bond the colonies within each colony there were many families and in each family group represented the tribal type of pocket where the love remained the core value. In the nuclei level the family was bound due to love bond a prevalent in the tribe and now additional inner core was developed where the family people had to interact with the other social groups developed (essentially the work place). It was the respect value found to have the bonding force. For a stable situation family became nuclei where love was vibrating and the inner core became the atom which was stable due to the respect. Harmony in the system was possible only when the atom and the nuclei are at their respective place or the values of love and respect kept vibrating in their own level.

It should also be remembered that in the tribal form love generated was from their inner self and for that reason it did not give them the opportunity to go into the intricacies but only knew of a force which came into existence to keep them safe and secure. It was only in the next stage of colonisation when the sanctity of love was realised and thus maintained at the core level of family.

Atomic level of humanity is the inner core in a big family; in inter family, kingdom, or the social circle where there are more than one unit involved to run the system. In such a place it was the respect value discovered important to maintain the harmony. The second swing towards the peak was the era when the respect was discovered and so was from their heart and the value was honoured.

It was also the time he was above the problem of his basic need and security because his mental faculty had started working more. There was devotion and dedication in the job whatever one was doing and hence there was the growth, which was shared. Persons involved in physical job were sharing their fruits with one who were involved in the mental work and visa-versa. It was the love value in a unit when extended in bigger units was termed respect. Sharing the fruits of their efforts in such environment was the cause of harmony in the system. This is represented as 'C' in the figure 3.1

Formation of outercore of mankind

In the next stage of civilisation it was the coalition of colonies, which gave the birth of nations as an acceptable stale format. There was plenty of advancement in logic sense by the time nation formation had started. This advancement had lead to urbanisation, industrialisation and having more of civic sense. There were sections for administration and security like activities. Due to the amalgamation of different pockets there where people with variance in customs and rituals at the inner core.

We see the changed system in 'D'of fig 3.1. We have nuclei, inner core and an outer core. The nucleus was the family and the relation where the love bond was essential and identical to tribal pockets. The inner core was the social pocket, culture pocket, farming sector, industrial area, administrative sector etc. at this level respect was responsible for smooth existence and the behaviour was identical to colonial form. For the harmony in the outer core which we also call as molecular level there were more than two units involved, where variation of custom and rituals were there it was the constitution which was followed.

If in one step earlier the respect was the force generated from the inner self it was actually realised. Subsequently it was utilised between the people who governed the nation and their citizen. The blend of love and respect to each other gave the formation of constitution. Advancement of urbanisation and industrialisation was taking place. People were working hard with dedication in their contributing of physical and mental work.

It was then a person doing both physical and mental activity realised a sense of satisfaction which people had been deriving earlier without realising it. On realising the satisfaction he analysed the behaviour and gave the credit to the mental faculty to cause the satisfaction and then he was bent upon minimising the physical labour of his activities that he was performing.

This is the break point on the day. The nation is the greatest single unit that can be considered. We are heading

FIGURE 3.2

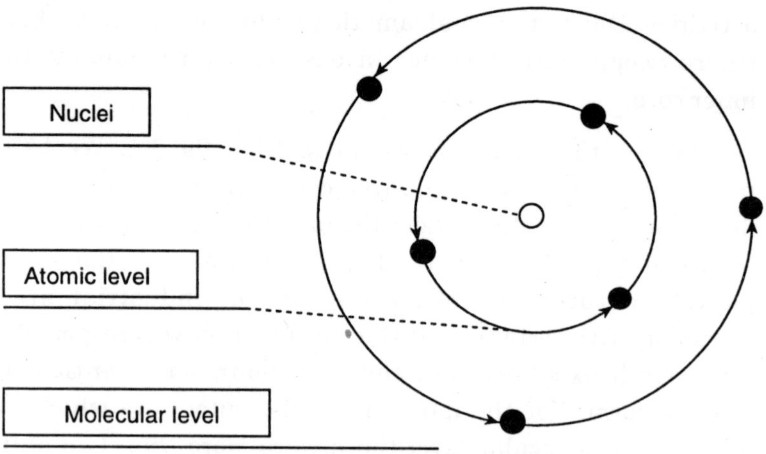

BASIC ELEMENT CONFIGURATION

towards E of figure 3.1 gradually. What is happening is different group of nations are subdividing human in few cultures from where they may break and again go the level 'A' which was the starting point.

This way we have discussed about the nuclei, inner core and the out core of mankind and give the term as *human element*. The human element has similarity with the basic element we know in science.

Stable element and its orientation

An element existing has essentially nuclei an inner core and an outer core. The outer core is the molecular level and the inner core is the atomic level. Any stable element has specific number of molecules orbiting in a specific orientation. Within a molecule the element has specific number of atoms orbiting in a specific orbit and has a nuclei at the core to make it live.

What happens if the orientation of the stable element is altered?

At the molecular level there are specific numbers of molecule. If the molecular orientation is change of the element the stability is changed and resultant there is a physical change observed. For example a plastic material which is very hard can change to softer (ductile) by this method or visa-versa. It is only the physical characteristic which is changed and the material remains the same. If the molecular orientation is more stream lined material is elastic and in haphazard form it becomes harder.

At the atomic level there are specific numbers of atoms orbiting in its stable sate. If the atom distribution is altered we observe a change which is chemical in nature. It may be higher or lower stability depending upon the addition or subtraction of atoms. The chemical change leads to the formation of element which has different name because it has the changed properties. For example radioactive material plutonium used for the energy in power plant after its life converts to a different element which becomes useless for that operation. In this case naturally the atomic substance release to give another lower form with different set of properties. In fact if the atomic orientation of any element if altered by some how it would lead to a formation of new element with very different properties.

The centre of the core has nuclei which is the binding source of the element. Nuclei cannot be disturbed. Destruction of nuclei would mean the destruction of the element when it would cease to exist and the substance would collapse.

HUMAN ELEMENT

Figure 3.3

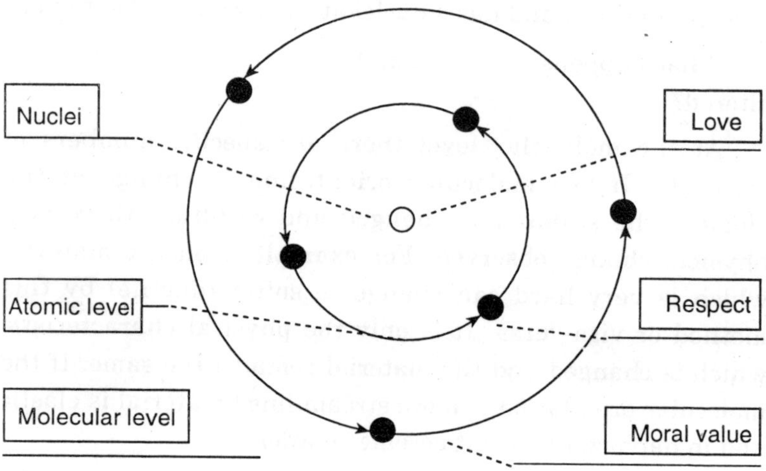

HUMAN ELEMENT CONFIGURATION

The civilisation has grown from tribal to colonial to national format. This growth has allowed adding the values forming different core of human element. At each level the basic values so generated had been nurtured and cared. If all the values are stable the human element is stable as in the case of any basic element. When the orientations of values are shifted the stability is disturbed and we come across with changed situation.

This situation gives us the opportunity to probe in details of humanity element which is of concern of present as well. We would be discussing further for a family as a unit with tribal-love value, organisation as a unit with colonial-respect value and nation as a unit with constitution-moral value as the ingredients together and separately which will allow us to draw a clear picture of what is happening in the world today and might reflect the demand of tomorrow.

In the human element the love is at the nuclei. It is the mental love at the nuclei , the strongest force to bind humanity. It is the love within a family, outside a family and al together love of human with human.

In the inner core as in the case of atoms the respect has to vibrate to maintain the harmony in a unit be it a family or organisation or a country or beyond the country. At the molecular level it is the constitution or the moral values that can maintain peace within each segment of human marked boundaries.

If all the three values keep vibrating in their respective place it would be an ideal situation of comfort and growth of mankind in all the units developed by him. It could be an ideal situation in the national format, which has been made till the day, and further growth of the mankind with is inevitable as the time flows. Economic and satisfying growth of a family depends upon only the three components present within them. An organisation be an industry or farming or any other social one can maintain appositive growth always if these three components are cared. Similarly a nation survives its boundary on keeping the three components vibrating in its place – but a human does not have a boundary limit. A person who understands love for others, respects others and follows morals is not bothered if he belongs to India, US or China.

Two important issues emerge here immediately are,

i. The time is not constant and stagnation is death. Hence the mankind has to grow further and not much time is left. Moving ahead would mean identifying another higher value and there remains only one which appears on the day which is beyond the national format and is the humanity. It is a concern by human for human.

ii. Rising in each step is more complicated as the variables have only increased on the way reaching there. If one section does think for humanity there are various different sections lying in different parts of the world, which are entangled, in the intermediate issues who are the bottleneck. These different units are with shifted orientation which requires more knowledge.

The second point relates the present state already existing.

- It could be the devil in us.
- Is there a simple solution?
- Do we know about the problem at the first place?

Knowledge is the first step and so if the problem is not known we have to identify. If the process of identification is started there would be a solution one day. We would further discuss about shifting values from their respective orientation in different units and sub units existing and how it is affecting the people. It could highlight a solution in the process.

Each of the three components viz. love; respect and moral value (or the constitution) are the upgraded mental status of the developed mind or developed human. The developed mind therefore is able to define a new value at an elevated state where as all the components were existing earlier within the system but were not required and so not seen as an independent function. With the development of mind the variance in the stable system and its instability is our subject but what is also of interest is that his elevated state had lot to change in the individual in his basic need as well. This change probably has confused some human who belong to the influencing stage of the world.

Shift of orientation in constitution (molecular level)

The largest unit defined is the national format and the value specified is moral value, which stands in the outer core of the human element. If the love is the strongest force, respect added is the superior mental status and if the constitution is added it calls for further superiority in the mental attitude. It is the mental freedom and positive approach which has brought human in the advanced stage and probably also taken further in few pockets. The history would tell that any type of external force is only able to elongate the time and becomes the barrier in the course of the forward progress. Countries, social groups, and individuals lagging cannot blame any one else but their position of existence their historical place today and the freedom they have in their country. We have to understand few words properly for knowing the change of orientation, which have a direct bearing on the subject.

A. Democratic behaviour

The national format is the biggest unit. In this context for the governing a nation it is only the democratic structure, which can lead to the shortest path for the progress. The democracy has to be understood by every citizen. It is the force when a citizen is ready to help and contribute what he can do for others. A government or the ruler cannot be said to be democratic if the citizen do not understand except when they are deprived of the minimum basic needs. A true democratic nation can sustain and survive and go beyond its boundary only when it is able to provide every citizen his or her basic need and simultaneously is able to shift the mental track of the people for positive contribution, which would ultimately cause them the satisfaction.

B. Physical element

The money had made the entrance in the society in the beginning of colonial format. The basis of creation was noble and was an effective tool to share between two sections of human that were not only doing different nature of work but also using different mental and physical energy in their part of the activities. It started with a barter system with exchange of one material to another material. People for their ease money was created as a medium of exchange. This money was a physical in character and important, its usage was related to the respect it is given. Till the time money was honoured for the purpose of exchange it was ok, but when it was not, its physical character was vastly exposed. Formation of any nation has a history and is associated with the struggle of their people to achieve it. Once the people achieve the freedom and come in the national format the meaning of constitution is realised by the key people and give the desired satisfaction. The satisfaction with time and generation is seen and enjoyed as a pleasure. When the pleasure word crops up in the mind there is an urge with a want of more. A human today within and out of the national boundaries have a misleading knowledge of satisfying pleasure and has an urge to fulfil it and wants to achieve it. If the evolved people are correct in diagnosing to achieve the satisfying pleasure in their mind it is the incorrect root they are applying. Satisfying pleasure is one step ahead in their mental frame and to achieve it he would need to have more civic sense than mere abiding constitution when he works for the humanity. The mankind has to reach as the next step forward. When it would happen? If at all it is quite far yet but would it happen at all is a concern of every good soul existing.

Reaching the state of such a pleasure is far but at present the pleasure is articulated as a commodity naming it as a thing for physical comfort and the reason for the elongation for the human path to progress. If money was seen as physical substance it became the tool to achieve pleasure but this was the actual intent and so the disturbance is created.

Refer figure 3.1 we would see that the constitution is in the outer core where the moral values should vibrate within the people and the ruler of a nation for a peaceful co-existence. On disturbing the constitution or the moral values from its path leads to physical change. This also changes the mental satisfaction for physical pleasure and displeasure in al the activities, which ultimately leads to mental corruption and inhuman instincts of physical nature. In such a situation yet if a nation wants to be peaceful it makes necessary for a ruler to make every citizen physically satisfied. At the superior level of mental status a human realises that physical satisfaction does not give him the contentment he has been searching.

1. Constitutions and the nation

Shifting of constitution from its path would mean changing of moral values. In a national format in such a situation the laws are amended to suit the prevailing situation. But the question is not of writing down a law and amending it. When the country gets independence it is associated with lot of human bonding elements such as sacrifice, togetherness, belief, faith towards a common goal for a free and strong independent nation. Till the feeling of integration of an independent nation is there not much of laws are required but as soon as independence is seen as an integral property of one self or a specific part of society within the first implication of shifting the values is observed.

Time is another factor of concern of the subject. The values generated up till the formation is a very gradual process and a hard earned effort of all. We also know now that the nation is the largest network of inter human relation developed and the equations formed till the day. In the freedom acquired the mental ability also is bound to progress could be in positive and negative direction. With negative mental ability rising and smaller segments (but essentially influential who are supposed to be the national leader political, economical etc) of the national network wanting to acquire independence in their own meaning tends the shift the constitution from its own path of vibration and want to do in a shortest time. This itself is breaking a natural law by their own people.

The moral values generated in ages if had the mental strength it cannot be speeded by few due to their fancy. If the subject is made an issue it could become an ego problem of those (influential part). The result is that assistance is taken of a physical force, which is the money. What it leads to? Is the corruption in the society or could be working more hours to acquire money rather than for peoples' benefit. Goal becomes the money and the time rides faster. Irony is that instead of trying to shorten the time the time shortens the life. With more working hours the inter human relation are further weakened.

What an ironical state! This has primarily generated a distinctly different culture in the world, which we term as western way from eastern, and the developing nation culture.

Human needs being same, how different culture can exist? Hence there is only one positive step ahead when people oversee the national boundary and entire human kingdom has one culture but it is very far dream if at all it has to happen.

C. Cultural difference:

In the chapter one we have described about the western and the eastern culture in details and the emergence of money power and the self (-ishness). But if money is so important for living how do we relate to physical element?

Whatever we get from nature it has a mental implication and whatever is made by human has physical implication.

Thousands of years ago when the civilisation had just started people use to cultivate grains for their requirement. The groups involved in the effort where sharing within themselves. With rise in the mental status when there were sections who were whole time devoted to give the benefit to the growers the sharing of the basic need was never an issue irrespective of their physical contribution being there or not. Later on with increase of more such creative groups in the colonial era barter system was started. This was the time when food habits were refined distinctively and they developed people wanted to have substance to get protein, vitamin etc. etc. in the form of fruits, vegetables, pulses meat. The farmers themselves did not grow all that they required and so all the sections be a grower or the person working in non farming area had to share the food for living.

Money was introduced in such a time with up gradation of the society and it was a mean by which sense of obligation may not generate in any section of the people. Harmony prevailed in the system because at that time there was deep strength of respect among each other. Till the time human needs were related to the natural things for food, cloth and shelter there was enough of contentment as these things were endless and what it required was the human effort to grow and grow.

With rise in logic sense and the technology when the utilisation of natural re-sources became equally important the same human started becoming dependent on coal, petroleum and minerals like things. The respect or the sanctity of the money was lowered once the human became dependent on such resources. Why?

As the natural sources are not endless and has a limit, the money did not have the strength to regenerate the source and keep intact the respect. Making himself dependent on such things (and then the mere thought that he could not live without it for any reason) was the primary reason to shift his mental cord to avail the man made requirement at any cost.

The basis of money for sharing the necessary good with no-obligation philosophy did not remain and it became the physical attraction and the power to the people involved in the mental activities with the negative leadership. Gradually the much loved money of today became the tool and the means to oblige to fulfil their requirement with newly dependent materials. Even today globally there is no shortage of money to feed the entire human community but the distribution is not proper.

In fact the money will be always sufficient for the basic need of whole human community but if it has become a tool for natural source related comforts in different walks of life it creates a snag. Definite (so called) comforts are the materialistic things which primarily are meant for those who are dedicated all the time for a cause of people or nature, for those who are dedicating the life for nation or the human community. The person finds it very difficult to measure his effort and relate to the extent of comfort that would really make him satisfying. It becomes difficult to even find if he can afford it and his aim becomes to use the tool (money) for exploitation. This exploitation could be even in the form of overworking when one is exerting more than he can do justice to himself for his ultimate generated desire. Apart each step of exploitation of any form is at the cost of some one in any part of the world. Such act is depriving of even of basic need to someone somewhere in the world knowingly or unknowingly.

In the mad race a person lying in the higher mental level (thinking to be educated and cultured) defining his own world of comfort often goes for exploitation with the basic aim to acquire more and more comfort. It is often too late for his experience to make him realise that it is the contentment that he was looking for rather than physical satisfaction. Many times one may even not have the knowledge about it. This exploitation of a person of higher mental ability definitely is the cause of deprivation of basic need of some person lying in the lower mental level somewhere in the world. Further this person at the lower level who could be satisfied and contended with the minimum basic need and would not ask for much from the life is forced to change his definition of contentment as food itself has become difficult for him.

Thus we see when the constitution (moral) is shifted form its orientation it brings the physical change in the human requirement and the outlook and he wanders in wilderness without the real aim for which the human was born. This phenomena can be easily observed by several changes that have been taking place in political system throughout the world situated at different levels of advancement in technology and society.

2. Constitution and the organisation

Within a nation a social group has been described as a human network which works for the people and thus the nation.

These social groups are such as farming, administration industries etc are seen as the colonies working within a nation generally satisfies the rule of colonial form of human civilisation. It is a smaller inter human network group and governed by few people similar to the kings. Within the organisation if we see with an open eye we would find a place of constitution in their framework playing an important part in the system.

We would discuss about the industrial colony, which is one of the important area of people concern, and also contribute to the national development. It would not be justified to explain the role of constitution in an industry of very small magnitude with few people working though it is a hidden element and essential one. Small or big organisations lay down certain laws, which are statutory by the government, but these laws are the theoretical part of the constitution. Actually from the point of view of human values there is something different more important to be known. The values have to flow necessary from both extreme high and low management. If the organisation has to survive and grow and work on the long term basis the element of constitution has to exist and followed by all. An organisation is truly professional only the constitution is there and every one follows it. Each segment of people are given their due respect and their share of contribution towards their work and every person works for the profit of an organisation.

Any organisation is an urban development work and the people working have to depend upon the money factor for their basic needs. When people get the mental security in an organisation they dedicate themselves in the job, and in such a situation a professional company would like to work on a rather lesser profit for its own and shared more by its people than having more profit for its own and sharing less with its people. Statistically if worked out former type would have overall less profit than the later type but it would have the strengthr to change the mental frame of the people, which would allow them to dedicate for the company to improve the quantity and the quality of the output resulting effectively more gain. Any statistic cannot show this in the beginning. Statistics is logic and logic cannot beat the values is the reason for it.

In the organisation set up what happens when the constitution is shifted from the orientation?

The effect is similar what we observed in the national framework. The aim becomes profit that is money and for gradual overall growth time appears to be hurdle. There is a sharp urge to acquire more money in the shortest time. To achieve the modified aim method utilised or visible is one by exploitation. Some start exploiting the people within the organisation some outside the organisation and some opt both. If for such results people work for very long hours they see only the money and in course of time move far away from the contentment which actually they aspire. In another situation a person finds him placed where he can not work for extended hours to generate money which has come in his mental track, he opts for corrupt practices. Here the act of being corrupt or to make corrupt may be appealing to the organisation as it directly shows the monetary benefit for the production to sell.

Corruption is a mental attitude which has a negative tilt. If money is very important thing and in the speeding age if one opts for corrupt practice and acquires good wealth and then thinks to lead a satisfied life he still would be not called a bad element. But definitely as it is a negative mental state it would not be so easy to get out of it. Majority of the cases he would be trapped and deviate from the main life goal in is maiden life he has got as a human being.

Stating again if the money can give basic need and the comforts, corruption can give fast bucks, all persons of an organisation if become corrupt and acquire sufficient wealth probably the practice they adopt would not be termed as corrupt practice but it could be understood as new developed culture. Such culture would have lots of snag and it would effect in quality of the products and consequently the organisation. Thus a small organisation well knowingly could opt for such system if they do not have a long term vision and are prepared for an early show down. A large organisation if follows such system it cannot sustain its name, fame and the respect. Therefore the shift of constitution makes a negative mental tilt which takes a person one step backward for satisfying life.

3. Constitution and family

What is the role of constitution in a family level? A family described is similar to a tribe where love value bond is the main strength where each member respects each other equally. Within a family constitution by no means can have a written down statement but finds its own importance where old and young all stay together. Constitution or moral values are made here on the basis of experience of members. The eldest in the family what ever his age is taken in confidence for any decision making. In such a system it is not necessary the eldest may have experience of every aspect of life and is always correct but to form a discipline the code of conduct is followed. In such a system where there is inter dependency of all the members every person has a share of contribution to put in for the positive growth of a family as a whole. Such system was prevalent in abundance in the early age of evolution. It exist today also in many parts of the world. If we analyse this system irrespective of any economic class people belong to each member has a tendency of sacrifice for his / her pleasure for others. The sense for sacrifice is stronger to maintain the constitution over anyone's' ego or for the physical pleasure which one is likely to lack.

In family when ego problem and physical comfort surface out sacrifice is seen as weakness rather than the strength. The sense of independence starts and leads in breaking the law. From the same family different groups crop up and what one says or listens to another member is different from what goes in their mind.

Shift of constitution from a family has the first effect in breaking the social norms to acquire independence, which further has all the open end for physical approach of life. His sense of love tends to be physical, his sense of comforts tends to be physical and thus the relation seems to be physical. His definition of comfort is the means by which he can satisfy himself physically. Love, which is the core value to bind a family, seems to change as a mere act of physical pleasure. The effect is so strong that even the art be a song or dance grabs the attention if physical exposure is present.

Shift of orientation in respect (atomic level)

In an element atoms are fixed and so their construction. The atoms have a specific orbital path which is maintained for a stable element. We have said further that if the atomic orientation is changed it becomes a different element as it results in the chemical change. In the humanity element the atomic core has similar behaviour. The respect value is responsible for its proper orientation. Respect was the strongest force to provide a stable colonial format.

The strength of the respect in the colonial system can be gauged by its role in different section of the society present. Colonial system had a king at the top who was not necessarily the most intelligent person in all the subjects. The king nevertheless had a fleet of intelligent people in a stable progressive colony in different walks of life and the king was only a coordinating agent. The king provided opportunity to all such intelligent individuals to fully utilise their mental skills, which could transform the benefit to the people till the bottom who were busy in physical activities for their contribution towards the kingdom. This process was not only helping the people economically but also trying to keep each segment and each person satisfied. If a person till the very bottom of the system could feel is contribution towards the common goal of running the kingdom it was because each section was given the respect needed.

Respect in the second largest value responsible for binding inter human network for a common goal. Past, present or future people unknowingly or knowingly have been doing constructive work and deriving pleasure. They have been responsible and have the key contribution for moving the humanity forward. Such people belong to different sections with different physical and mental capabilities and thus different working on different fields but derived satisfaction remains the same in all of them. If the satisfaction is in doing, contentment is in thinking, and the pleasure is in performing both. Persons who have been deriving such satisfaction, contentment and the pleasure yield the fruits for others in the form of food, clothing, shelter, guidance peace etc.

Whether it is farming generating the food for the body for others or be an art in the form of music, dance, painting etc generating food for the thought or could be scientific development sharing ones part increases the mental level along with the satisfaction. The satisfaction achieved in each such case is two folds

- one for achieving the goals and
- other for the sense of their contribution in sharing with others.

A music composer may not have a direct link with the

farmer but they also are interdependent on each other for the continuity of their sound and peaceful life. The interdependency is of human to human and by that only the development of societies has taken place. Today each activity be the tiniest one has been explored by the researchers to give a full scape dimensions and thus generating endless avenues. Till any avenue is given its due respect there is sharp positive development in that area but when any segment of the society tries to shift the respect value the foremost deviation affects the mental approach. It happens, as one has to suddenly come out from the deep well of contentment and has to chase a person who has destroyed his peace and it results instinctively showing his self-respect. EGO if aroused it is difficult to say how many people can come back to their original state.

1. Respect and the nation

A nation is a sovereign state with its own law of the land to rule but essentially consist of people belonging of many religions of different cultures and traditions. With societies formation and different segments given different roles there has been further subdivision of classes. The different religions which relates to the self discipline and different classes, which relates to social discipline were thus formed. Each individual and each social segment had its own role to play for moving the system forward and it was possible only when due respect was given to all the individuals or the groups.

The aim of a nation is to progress which implies the progress of all the individuals. But the progress is not the economic factor alone. The progress would mean up gradation of all in their mental status, improvement in thinking and adding value in their life and further applying their skills for the benefit for one another. There is a great difference in the work allotted to different segments of society and it could be gauged from the physical and mental activities required to carry out their job. Each of these segments requires equal respect without creating any sort of complex situation. Only a positive attitude in thinking and doing can be a source to carry out the job and still command the respect.

In the Mahabharat epic societies are divided in four classes as Brahmins, Kshatryias, Vanijyas and Shudras. It was not the division for giving any more respect to some or disrespecting any class but had the positive implication in doing so. As per the need of the society and to fulfil the ego of the people the entire society was sub divided according to their mental capabilities. The highest capability of the mind were termed as Brahmin (intellectuals) and accordingly given the role of uplifting the knowledge of the people and thus the society. A little less mental capability but with enormous skills were the Kshatryias (warriors) for the adventurous jobs and safe guard the society from unwanted forces. Next in descending order of mental capabilities were Vanijya (Merchant) were given the role for the distribution of the basic need to the society. The last but not the least in order were Shudras (lowest class) with less mental capability were allocated for cleaning the environment to maintain hygienic conditions of the society. This gradation was made not for any separation of classes but was for human to chose their slot with their mental capabilities and join hand for working or contributing their part to the society.

It is equally important to understand the basic need of each group, which was not similar. The eating habits and the food requirement to have sense of fulfilment and maintain their health and continue doing their chorus to help the society has relevance to their mental capabilities. People with very less mental capabilities in the shudra category are capable to survive even if they have to work in an unhealthy environment and require more and cruder food for his body nourishment. For this reason they were chosen for maintaining the hygienic condition for the rest. On the other hand a Brahmin with a very high mental aptitude needed much refined and lesser food for his body nourishment and for activating his creative skills. A Brahmin thus was given the charge for educating the society, to develop the skills in human for the up-liftment of values and thus the mental level of the rest. A person with mental attitude of former if placed in the job of later or visa-versa would be a failure.

The four categories are not any distinct classes for distinguishing a family or a group in the society. A person belonging to lower mental level could be in shudra category and could have adopted the work to suit it but when one such person is able to lift his / her mental aptitude he / she would automatically come in the next higher defined class which has a different role to play for the society. This is an ideal situation and the philosophy would be applicable when person of each class are given their due respect and in turn such people respect their work assigned and fine the contentment. The money is a man made thing and is of physical nature. The money has the respect only till each segment is given their due respect. With the lust of money if any segment opted to disrespect others and his work he would lose the respect. Even if such person generated wealth and became above his basic need (form his own point of view) he has no option other than demanding the respect, which he has broken. This would amount to the shifting of respect value from its orientation and would lead to inter human rivalry resulting a negative seed in their mind ending up in anti human tactics of violence.

Change in atomic level leads to a change of chemical in nature with the resultant element of absolutely different properties. Similarly change in the respect value changes the mental attitude towards the negative side. The negative mind starts becoming dominating in all the fields. The impact may or may not be apparently visible in a wide national network but the fact that the stable independent nation formation has been the cause of dedicated people who have followed the positive path for their country, adhered and enriched certain values in the process. When such dedicated people are over shadowed by the negative leaders there remains no one to guide and make realise to the new active lot about the national feeling which was essential to sustain as a growing nation. The process gradually changes the mentality of the major chunk of the people towards the unwanted negative side, which delays and defers the progress of the country.

2. Respect and the organisation

Within a national framework respect value has been the prime force in the stable organisational system. The organisation could be farming, industry or any other social part. The system is colonial type with much simpler and smaller goals. As the king the organisational head forms the rule with the objective for people to do a piece of job such that as an end result the organisation is able to produce goods. The attempt is that each person's work profile could be quantified in measurable units of time and return they are given with a specified quantity of money.

The parameters of time and quantity are man made measures for their disciplinary consideration. Such system when formed it was in line to the philosophy where one can gauge the respect for his contribution for the organisation. The contribution of people would be of physical and mental in varying proportion where all have to respect the organisation, which is their feeding end.

For effective contribution towards the organisation it is important each of them respect their work and of course it goes without saying it would mean giving respect to each member as in a happy family. Measure of time has great value imbedded within. It has an absolute dimension in itself. Time gone is time gone and can never be recovered. In the scientific age scientist have tried to catch the time by various method of speeding the life. It is difficult to understand what people have achieved by speeding the life when the end goals have been material related and are speeding has been at the cost of something invaluable.

An organisation is generally not a charitable one and so the end goal is connected to the money, profit for the body. Its simultaneously important role is to lift the mental frame, which would be understood easily. There is a threshold limit of a human speed, which can bind him in the frame of respect. When and where the threshold limit is crossed it is at the cost of respect in one or another form. Giving more money to form a new standard in quantum of output is adopted system which is a motivating tool. Crossing a threshold limit would mean disrespecting the product if focus is made in quantity for the production or setting parameters beyond the optimum level forcing one again to over see the quality or create a chose in the working mind. Such a situation would have a tendency to generate fear in himself and a sense of insecurity would loom in persons mind. The negative implication has allowed create unions, association and forums in the organisation. Formation of cohesion platform is the straight indication of negative implication and by this time the respect also turns physical character and loses its shine.

May be another organisation understands about the standard and the quality and when it sees the crack in the system because of speeding the life it goes more scientific and utilises the machine instead of human. The replacement of human by machine has either of the following implication.

i. If the organisation is small it might make people out of job and cultivate a sense of insecurity.

ii. If the organisation is big and starts giving much more profit and if the profit is shared by all (operating professionally) in such situation it would cause an insecurity of the smaller or other competitors operating un professionally. Within such profitable venture there is a chance the sharing of profit could add extra money to a section of people who actually do not require or cannot digest. Result is that such person start looking for unimaginable comfort which they are not intended for the basic contentment. There are chances of missing the opportunity for the realisation or delaying it when the comfort and pleasure are looked as an end rather than the contentment.

Thus deviation of respect from its orientation generates a negative line of thinking, which could result a closure of unit, sacking of people or enjoying the extra pleasure, and comfort which one is not intended to do.

Administrative set up or personnel department is there to control an organisation. If we recall the initial human development the administrative traits were generated from the natural negative instinct and so this department has the negative behaviour and so the end result is again negative. With time and knowledge for this reason to counter the negativity, organisation have started or termed the word of human resources, which should work, on human logics and behaviour to and the positive instinct. Such moves can be effective only when the respect is restored in all the individuals between themselves and towards the organisation as a unit.

Time parameter is man-made measure and the speed of life we have discussed is a natural way that cannot be quantified and so realisation of time becomes important from the point of view of its value. It could infer that the positive growth could be gradual and in many instances slower than desired or achieved. It could be positive if the extent of quantifiable comforts with the lower end of section are lower and are satisfied and it would also amount of larger section being satisfied and enjoy the basic comforts that deserve. It should be also understood that with time and up gradation the definition of individual requirement changes and does not remain fixed. This way a positive mental track and creativity can be inducted which could cause to all individual to respect the work, respect the material and respect another human being.

Let us observe the implication of deviation of respect and the mental frame in another set of social unit. In the process of human evolution the roles of women was made within a family and to look after all the chores at home. If physical job assigned were to cook and do the household jobs the mental job was given to bring up the children and develop for tomorrow's society. It still remains the assigned task in many parts of the world. We should also not forget that women were the first who inspired the real meaning of mental love from where the civilisation had started. And therefore they were given a great responsibility and by no means a small and unaccountable roll to play in the society.

With passage of time and the advancement of values and the technology over all 'mental frame' of all have gone up. In such a situation respect may not be only the shortest path for contentment and would require additional value.

What happens in a social system if one goes ahead in manipulation of skills to cut certain social norms by showing disrespect?

The consequence is negative for human and the civilisation. Since ages women have been doing all sorts of jobs and have possessed the leadership qualities in many cases. In the present world where prime force is human value if one is doing creative and constructive work one is deriving a pleasure en-route to contentment irrespective the doer is man or woman. Even such a recognised woman would not deny the role given to the women in the society and would not speak for the equality. They would know that there had never been any un equality.

Why should a woman be as a man and not as a woman?

May be such an issue of liberation and equality allow few to get renown and find some followers to make them leader but that only allows to break the harmony in the society. It is only the breaking of natural law generated with time and experience at the cost of respect, which they do not understand.

The issue of women liberation and equality is very big and of great importance. A woman and a man make a unit to run the civilisation. The half of the world population is of women and so how there can be inequality. A comparative line is drawn only to hurt oneself. In a gradual progression of mankind certain norms were laid for both men and women and were for the fulfilment of both. Each sex had the mental security in performing the assigned task. Both had the scope of deriving the contentment and for that respect for each other was the most essential part of a society.

It does not mean that a woman is only to bear a child and look after the family. A constructive person can find a useful time for anything. And it all starts like this

– The situation of equality starts where most of the physical job are replaced by the machines. This is the first point where the norms are disrespected and the extra time available which was intended for physical job is not vested in some physical form and thus the equilibrium is shifted. A typical physical and mental work together gives the satisfaction towards the contentment to a person of a normal mental frame which varies widely person to person. Now if physical work are deleted and one wants to be contended one would have to either replace that time with some physical constructive activity or go in the higher mental frame where thinking of humanity would come itself and consequently there would be no issue of equality at all. Once more thus we see that shift of the respect value alters the mental frame in the negative direction leading to different evil and disturbance.

3. Respect and the family

The smallest social unit is a family and to run it smoothly element of constitution and respect are required. It being the primary unit in our theory of mankind the core value binding is love but with the increase of mental frame of the people respect has its own important role to play. This primary unit is of most importance not only to itself but to the social, national and above all the universe. The essence of its formation is love but the social acceptance of the method at higher mental frame is for inter relation of people where family word can extend to limitless end.

Smallest family unit would comprise of parents, husband-wife and children and they make three generations. In the olden times when little was known about the global consequence people had many children and the value was imbedded within them. (This is to remind the readers that where the respect was not given due they could have delayed the progress in the path of their evolution and do not play a significant role in the context) Probably with more people within the unit they had the opportunity to live with different types of mind and knew or learnt to adjust in living with them. If the head of the family had the satisfaction as the leader of the group to fulfil his ego each of the children and so many companions to make an idea for any decision. This not only led to progress ahead but also taught them the patience attitude. To hear against one way or to see against one wish gave them different point of views. The process enabled them to enrich themselves.

With advancement of basic knowledge and the awareness of his logic and the concern of the health and future they had fewer children but mere knowledge can not lead to the realisation. The difference between the earlier and the later case was that when family was very big the child had the opportunity to realise by their brothers and sisters (in the smallest circle) and it was associated with the sense of sacrifice the act which was responsible to generate patience which in turn allowed them to enrich the respect between them for the parents. In the later case with fewer children there could be two probabilities,

- If one is in the similar mental frame it becomes important to be closer with more like kinded people in the society and realise the issue rather than know a single point of view in any subject.
- Or to raise one mental frame where every act need not be realised only by the physical act. It is the state of mental level where a person with a needle prick can realise the pain when hurt with a dagger.

If a person or a child as in the above case does not belong to any of the mental frame he may not have the actual sense of realisation and in such a case one cannot have the knowledge of respect and could disrespect the family members. The first attack on the respect by such a person is on the parents and subsequently on the society. The first question generated in a person when the respect is dislocated is *why?* To all the norms laid down and are followed blindly by the society.

Why I should agree with them? Why should I follow them? Why should I work for them? And so on.

The generation of word 'why' in such a place makes the mental shift and the child does not hesitate to infer that their parent's role has been only to bring them in this world. Any parent would support a child till he could stand independently on his own. He thinks its his duty and tries to enrich his experience in the child's life. He does so because he has a certain amount of respect for the child and not for what he wants in return. But in the situation if the respect is not returned back to the parents the child loses the one lifetime opportunity about the value that he can gain by the experience.

As far as the parent – child relation is concerned the respect value cannot be taken out in absolute term due to the natural laid procedures. It is for the survival of their species or their class as they could think parents have to care for their children no matter whatever sacrifice they have to make. The children are brought up and guided by parents till a certain age however parents cannot disown them mentally. In the case of children in the worst case if one disowns his parents physically it is possible that one realises the act of the disrespect except it could be too late to be pardoned. The mental strings cannot be broken so easily even if the physical acts show that way.

The relation between man and woman has altogether a different sort to tell and a different basis to work. Men and women are two independent persons with an independent identity. Marriage of the two has a great significance in our society and the civilisation. Wedding could have been the stating point of human civilisation and the most important element between them to tie up is the faith, trust respect for each other.

The faith is the respect of our concern. Gradual experience made them realise that two of them form a unit and thus two units become half to form a complete unit. Each of them agree to share good and bad, happy and sad moments together and thus share in providing the mental security to each other. Till the faith is between them the combination of physical effort and the mental security, it so works that with the feeling of comfort both become dependent on each other. This is only a way that the harmony can prevail. Being dependent both the persons get the opportunity to fulfil their ego for their part of importance if it exists. The man and the woman come from two different families with their own identity and have a reason to live together happily and thus this relation helps in fact bringing them closest both physically as well as mentally *but* till the faith is existing between them. If a crack is generated in the faith between them the self identity and the ego surfaces out and the question crops up of *why. Why am I so dependent on the other?* The comfort and the pleasure, which was being derived from the dependence, are hampered.

So if the respect in such case is shifted form the stable axis the mental security of either partner is loosened and the attack is on the relation between them. The situation can have two different ends,

i. It can either lead to a broken life then after or

ii. One could seek an independent living when the definition of comfort itself changes for them. They get comfort only if they can spread the importance of respect for every human.

Such isolated cases can help restore the respect in this world. On the other side if the meaning of respect were not realised by a large chunk of people how would the civilisation continue?

Thus when the respect value be in the national unit of an organisation as a unit or a family shifts from the stable axis there is a change in the mental attitude which is similar to change in the element in the atomic level where we observe the change in chemical properties.

Why we relate the mental change as the chemical change is for the reason that human physical body is like a chemical engineering set up and whatever the reactions happening has a direct bearing in the mental organ. The change in the mental frame from the proper orientation causes the negativity in the mind and thus the thinking resulting in action. Such chemical change could not only harm one self but could influence the surrounding environment even more.

Shift of orientation in love (the nuclei)

If the nucleus is eliminated from an element the element collapses or cease to exist. May be it is not possible practically or is difficult for human to visualise today. Similar is the role of love value in the humanity element. Eliminate the love and the humanity collapses. May be human can not visualise this also but this state has to be realised much in advance for the progress of our civilisation before one finds that the time becomes the limiting factor.

Love is such a basic ingredient that even the animals understand it to run their race. It was the human who invented as a bond and the logics started. In the process of human evolution it was the tribal format where the human developed the knowledge of love. They knew the importance of this value and for that they progressed further. If the love were taken out from their path they would have been in animal cadre and so we. If the love were taken out from the animals the survival of the race would cease to grow.

Love has its unique role to play not in the humanity alone but the universe. We have seen earlier that for more than two units to exist in harmony constitution or moral value is essential, for two units to exist in harmony respect value is essential and where there is only one unit love is the prime force to mere exist. The one, two or more units could be one living being could be a family, could be a society or an organisation or nation or any part of our segment whatever term we use.

The love is major value for a self itself, to exist it has its importance in any bigger segment which is only the accumulation of human and increased numbers or unit that are forming other segments. Therefore in each enlarged segment love still remains the hidden value very necessary for that group to exist.

Going above the self in the present mankind state by the theory a family is the smallest unit. In terms of value it is correlated to the one with tribal format. The role of love can be understood very easily in a family. It has similar role in an organisational and national set up where it's meaning could be further broadened. There is physical and mental part of every step of mankind, which has brought up till the present stage. With time the proportion of physical and mental are changing but both exist.

i. In a family the physical satisfaction is in the form of the feeling of touch.

ii. In the organisation the physical love is in the form of basic needs one is deriving

iii. In the national system it has the importance in feeling secure.

The mental love, which has to grow stronger in all the section including the self, is the state where a person realises the value and the importance of humanity and starts becoming more logical. In each stable system mental love exists and has to grow stronger to prosper in the basic level.

But in today's world with varying state of evolution and thus varying degree of mental frame existing there could not be a place where singly love is the acting force. The situation is enriched with varying degree of the other values described earlier. In such a situation if a person thinks that he is deprived of human values, he has lost the respect there are two strong probabilities ahead with the basic value of love which would make or break his life.

ii. In one of the instance he would enhance the lost love by interacting more with the people and thus contributing a positive construction for the people as a result finding a solace. With time he would generate the respect and the human values in a specific place of the society.

iii. In another case if one has not understood the lost love the person might have an aimless time which would prompt him to finish one self which is a disastrous act. If he does not finish himself he might be trapped with some physical disorder, which again would lead him to end the life.

The importance of the love value can be judged in the self independent feeling which as engulfed in a western culture and all also the others following the rule. It is the culture where dependency on material and money is on extreme. In acquiring material he his ready to shift from the constitution which is a path of human code of conduct for his convenience, if he realises so further there is an urge for demanding respect by money power. These are the physical changes, which are utilised for fulfilling his false ego, and what ever he does is at the cost of hurting the basic value of love within one self and the society or any of the larger group of the format of the civilisation. This is the cause, which breaks the human social bonds of parent - child or husband - wife. In such a situation the way out for the contentment are few.

i. To dedicate the left over life selflessly for other humans

ii. If he does not have the ability or due to the circumstance available he cannot come closer to the human community he could start loving the nature. Nature is available everywhere except one has to have the inclination for the attachment toward it. It could be for saving a virgin piece of land where human devastation has not started or restoring a piece of land, which has been humanly mutilated for his comfort.

iii. There is another avenue where one has to lift oneself in the spiritual level where all the love has to be showered to the supreme power (God) in whatever shape one can visualise.

As love value is essential for a single unit it is essential for every self to have it at the first place for mere existing to associate other values in the system. It is every one's personal property where he has the right to acquire. The system works when love of every individual in the group combines to give the sum of the love to all. This is to say if two persons possess one unit of love each and when the meet and share what each get is two unit of love. On the other hand if one is starved of love and interacts with another he would reduce the love ingredient in the other person also.

If a lost love can break a family which has been the strongest ever made for running the civilisation at the higher ladder of social format or at the national format bigger disaster can happen.

In the social level or the organisational level the love value is associated with the basic need. The surety of basic need allows one to contribute both physically and mentally for the people or for the organisation and simultaneously allows him to run his family also.

In the national system love is attached with the security one expects form his country. If the security of individual is in peril the nation can also break.

Thus we see that slight deviation of love form its stable axis starts causing a break in a persons' own life or has a tendency to break the other stable system of organisations and the nations.

CHAPTER 4

FUTURE WORLD AND THE MENTAL FRAME

The mental frame or the mental level word has been coined in this chapter, which should be understood properly. The mental frame of any human being is a status of a mind, which has a specific requirement for achieving him / (her) the satisfaction as understood by a person. The satisfaction is achieved by the sum of the activities carried out of physical nature to consume his physicals energy and the mental nature consuming the mental energy. The understanding of mental frame is very important because ingredient for satisfaction even for the basic need defers for different mental frames and thus varies in all human beings. We would not go in much detail at an individual level but such mental frame can also be defined for the higher units formed by human and identify the basic ingredients required for its stability. Nevertheless it is important to know the following,

i. Lowest mental frame is that of people staying very closely to the animals. It is their natural evolution state inherited from the chain of the circumstances and does not mean not make them inferior.

ii. Once there is a rise in a mental frame of any unit it cannot reduce. Either it would stagnate or rise only. Hence improvement has to be there, it could be slow or fast and requires effort.

iii. Each mental frame has a different way for his approach to the individual life or for the others. Rising in mental frame if said to be refined method it is at the cost of losing something.

iv. Satisfaction could be desired goal till a specific mental frame but it is the contentment which is the ultimate desired goal knowingly or unknowingly of any unit existing. This is for a simple reason that satisfaction has an end and is time bound or short-lived thing where as the continuation search of satisfaction is the contentment. Contentment is continuous and endless.

It is also important to make understand the readers that in the context of higher society of family or organisation or nation we relate the incident, which pertains the message to be imparted, which could have larger bearing on the system or the society. Either we talk of the ideal situation, which it should be or discuss on the situation causing the deviation and thus the repercussions that tends to break the system. The majority could be lying in between who are the safe followers on either side of making and breaking system. They do not form important for a simple reason that the person or any unit responsible for going up in the ladder of humanity or breaking the system are the leaders and are of our concern.

Mental frame of a bigger unit of our system:

A nation is highest level of recognised unit in the humanity. The nation would have people with varying composition in religion, caste and with varying state of the evolution. It has one head as per their constitution and the nations working varies as autocratic, democratic, communist and so on. Even if there is one assign leader of the nation any decision pertaining to the nation or for their people is taken jointly by a group for the assigned function. The decisions that are the policy matters are responsible to guide the country in a definite direction. The direction could be towards positive growth of the path that delays the growth. Accordingly the nations can be assigned with a mental frame and has the reflection of her future path whether the decision is taken by a group or by any individual. A nation may have people of different mental state in the context of the humanity evolution and would have with varying degree of logic sense. However the leader or leaders with their collective policies would also indicate the national state in terms of its placement in humanity and logic sense. It can not be that every one is satisfied but definitely from a national point of view a positive growth could be gauged if policies are made honestly that helps the people and from the other perspective average people do not exploit and thus the minimum gain goes to the person in the lowest ladder. If this could be a hypothetical state country by en large if develops a culture it would be not impossible.

An organisation which is a smaller unit operating on colonial function has a king (type) leader with their supporting team for running the show. Like the nation the policy could be for the positive growth or with delayed tactics for the organisation and the people working in it. The policy could be formed by the leader or by the group the organisational status with its functioning would indicate its place in mental frame as an organisation. Even though the people working in the organisation could be of much higher or lower mental frame at the individual level the mental frame of the organisation is not the average mental frame of the people and it can not be said of the leader as well. The positive growth could be observed with the quality of the product and the services and thus depends on the policies made by the leaders and the execution done by the entire force. The energy put by the people continuously would also depend upon the work satisfaction, the comfort feeling on the basic need at the individual level and thus the culture developed in the organisation.

In both of the cases we find that it the unit concern has a

positive growth in the humanity level it would amount to develop typically a separate culture. We call it a culture because it would make every person of that unit (national or organisational level) would participate from their level to maintain irrespective of the individual mental frame. By doing so a person who is relatively in the lower mental ladder is able to understand his basic need, is focused on his part of work and in the process lifts his mental frame at the individual level which helps to provide the contentment in the act.

Today United Nation Development programme prepares Humanity Development Index to grade the condition of a country. The parameters considered are like per capita income, education level, health care and life expectancy. It's a good attempt but can be useful if the experience of the countries in the top can be given to the lower ones such that the difference could be narrowed down. A good living from the above measure is possible if the country has good economy but it cannot sustain unless the culture is developed which gives the contentment. Any amount of money or the material can provide satisfaction but cannot provide contentment. Without achieving the contentment the satisfaction would have the dead end, as it would lead to the stagnation of the mental frame.

On the other hand there are economically poor countries who at this stage need much economic satisfaction and contentment at present. They find difficulty in acquiring the minimum resources available in abundance else where in the world. Can these two and all other intermediate stages be connected for the betterment of the human community irrespective of their placement in this world?

It is the clash between the values and logic sense of a nation that is contributing the slow down of the progress or preventing the positive growth forward as a whole.

The world today is distributed in the national format. There are nations with very small territory and nations with very large territory. There are nations with different type of governance. Some nations have many cultures and religions imbedded and some have very few. Some have very openness where as some are very conservative. Some care for others where as some cannot care for them selves. Some have huge natural resources but are not high on economical status where as some have very few natural resources still dictate the world on economics. Some appear politically strong and some are strong where as some appear politically weak where as they have potential beyond it appears.

Two critical stages existing today are,

i. Nations falling in the lowest level of humanity development and have enough known scope for advancement by the experience of the nations already passed that stage. They find it difficult and require the assistance of the developed nations.

ii. There are nations, which fall in the highest ladder of human development. Some have crossed the satisfaction stage (in the national format) and are probing for the next climb.

Rest all the remaining nations are in between these two states. They could simply follow the path found by the nations ahead or could bring the deviation in positive or negative side.

The present world state is considered as post-colonial era but in our humanity graph that is not the correct nomenclature. There are several big and small nations advanced and not so advanced nations that still have the colonial structure. The colonial structure decides the mental frame and the hence the necessary value required for stability can be judged. The logic sense, which relates to the scientific advancement to give comfort also plays equally important role. The logic sense or the scientific advancement of a nation has following probabilities,

i. A nation could be on a having a higher logic sense from a political point of view. It would mean a nation appears to be in an advanced scientific state but the comfort actually does not reach to the minimum required people and so what appears is illusion. Such illusion also would mean the absence of liberal or democratic structure in a country where the communication would be far unclear to the outside world. There could be positive or negative step further as following,

a. In a positive step the country has to realise the need of the mass and liberalisation could help to evaluate the status on value which could help to understand that system followed till now is of colonial format and thus to rise to the national format they have to have a constitution (not the theoretical piece of written statement) but the political climate for the countrymen. It would boil down to provide a system structured so that the benefit reaches till the bottom of the system. It is also important to know that if larger section of people are still under colonial format unknowingly their requirement of comforts are unreal. By this we mean that in such existing structure if logic sense was appearing high probably the scientific comfort was with the hands who did not require where as in the same country the one who could be requiring were depriving of it. Alteration of democratic system is only the solution but it would cause lot of internal turmoil because of the imbalances existing. It could require a help of other nation on actual national format and would take time and generations to come in a stable system.

b. In a negative step the imbalances of money, comfort and the power in the hand of people who are not the true requirement could find themselves influential with the nations of similar or lower mental stage for a tie up. The tie up would be for a personnel individual benefit and would lead to chaos or civil war, internal unrest or also could break the nation.

ii. In another case a nation could be advanced in values and also advanced in logic sense but still operating in a colonial format. In such case even if the people are above basic need and theoretically satisfied, it could be a temporary mental state in isolation. It is the contentment, which is the final goal, and the nation would face mental crises to overcome and come to the next step. For the next step here again nothing can be done in isolation and what would be required is the peoples' contribution to the outside world. Here there are again a positive and a negative sides that could follow as,

a. The nation where most of the people are satisfied from the basic need would mean that they would have a culture to signify the satisfaction to the world. Their willingness to spread the culture beyond the country us the direct forward positive step. In an individual situation a spiritual could be way, which means to be more powerful mentally, and lesser interest on physical way of life. On the national format rising higher in value is the ladder of humanity. Such nation would find contentment in associating and helping other nations and the people to lift from their lower mental state by full participation even if it is at the cost of physical discomfort, which does not matter much.

b. On the negative step probably the nation would try to disconnect itself from the other world in the lower mental state. We are satisfied and do not want to hinder the peace prevailing could be political thought. It could work for few generations but automatically lead to discomfort. If they donot rise up in the mental frame the degradation could be seen in the physical form. The lust of life in physical form could be seen more prominent in the section of people rising in the nation and could mislead them in balancing the value and logic sense and thus lead to disaster.

To draw an analogy of different nations on the basis of above hypothesis the whole spectrum can be framed in general format on the following basic background of the theory:

1. Lowest mental section is that of the animals where only natural instinct exist for survival and keeping the race alive.
2. Next level of mental state belongs to the tribal format where the love was the core value invented.
3. Next above is the colonial format mental level where the core value generated was respect.
4. Above this mental level relates to the national format where the core value identified is moral value.
5. Final step above is the mental level of humanity. As a section it is still to be formed. It could be observed in sections but has to emerge as a force ahead.

It would be important to make aware our good reader that we are referring only the positive movement ahead responsible for the rise in humanity.

Placing the details in a tabular form:

Column-I	**Column-II**	**Column-III**	**Column-IV**	**Column-V**
Reference level	Assigned group by the hypothesis	Existing related section	Core value required	Ultimate Goal
M 5	Culture	Humanity	Humanity	Contentment
M 4	Nations	International organisation	Moral value	Contentment
M 3	Colonies	Social group	Respect	Contentment
M 2	Tribes	Family	Love	Contentment
M 1	Animal survival	-	Basic instinct	Survival of species

Column V: The ultimate goal: Is a hypothetical word in general terms for the reason that majority of the human belong in the follower group but essentially it is the ingredient which one is trying to discover in ones one life span in different ways and different experience. Infinite experiences are going on different levels for a same goal, which is contentment.

Why we call contentment as a final goal has been described earlier is for the reason it is endless. Contentment is the state with positive movement that keeps showing the path ahead.

Column IV: Even when we call contentment as unending goal the core value is defined which indirectly limits for the specific unit following in that category. What we mean here is the core value itself is sufficient for the relevant unit to derive satisfaction.

1. Either the unit would not move ahead substantially ahead in a short time and keep deriving contentment in the process or
2. If the unit were in the threshold of crossing the limit it would belong to the next higher level.

Column III: Are the examples of the existing units belonging to the mental levels but does not limit. In fact any unit from an individual to any larger group can be fitted and examined on the chart.

Column II: Is the defined state of the stable format where relevant values were recognised according to the theory.

M-1 is the lowest mental frame where survival and the basic need are enough for the contentment. None human being today belongs to this category.

M-2 originally belongs to tribal system. Today it is relevant to small family units where love value is enough for the contentment.

M-3 belongs to the colonial system. Today it has relevance to the social units, organisation and even with many countries.

M-4 belongs to the national format where moral value is the route for contentment. Very large organisation also would fall in this category for their route for contentment.

M-5 is the culture of a large segment of human comprising of multi nations and religions as one block. The world is gradually proceeding towards it. It consists in broken form and has yet to acquire a recognised format. This is the format where all individuals irrespective of their country would work for the human of this world. Their route of contentment is humanity.

All these values have significance if observed in one upward direction but does not happen *in absence of knowledge for the goal of contentment or if the mental frame for any reason is stagnant or rising very slow the sense of discomfort starts building.* The values are the first victim and are hurt by various methods.

There is another variable playing the part to confuse different units. Irrespective of mental frame of a unit is stagnant or rising slowly the scientific development around the unit adds the logic and ultimately affects the speed of life of the unit. It also tends to make a unit independent of another unit but in that course ends up making dependent on the material or the natural source.

Logic sense if is defined a means to provide a physical comfort it becomes very important for one to know where the unit or any individual belongs and how much of physical comfort is required. This need to be gauged by the exertion put in the mental sector in carrying out the *positive* activities. This is to say that if a unit belongs to a mental frame M-3 and tries to measure its comfort of higher level it would amount to create imbalance in the system. Either the unit has to raise the mental frame, which cannot be done by a magic wand, or put restrain in the logic sense. It is only a different route one would require than one is adopting and if applied with the true spirit the passage would become clear with time automatically. The unit would meet hardships, which only have to be seen as challenges to overcome successfully without any short cut. Largest unit existing today is the nation. Be a nation or any organisation it has human with varying degree of mental frames in the individual level. The leader or the head is generally be assumed to give the indication about the general mental frame of a stable nation or organisation where it would be said the leader at the higher mental level is able to understand the need of his countrymen and making suitable policies to suit them. If the mental frame of the leader itself is not the best and clashes with the (higer) logic sense it cannot give the best. Highest position would get the best comforts which should not mistaken as their necessity. The simplest measure is to evaluate if one demands or commands. Unit head demanding comforts would also demand respect, demand love and would certainly miss the moral value and end up in clashing within his country or with the other country.

Testing of hypothesis

Below is the list of examples of some important countries and the events which we would try to put them in our hypothesis and find out what does the situation indicates

The events were news items and are more than 15 years old. In fact the news items were of great importance then and sorted out in 1989 when the essay was written for the first time.

We would take up each of these events with the description of the origin of the country in the subsequent part of 'Mental Theory And The Nation'.

1. Release of apartheid leader Mr. Nelson Mandela.
2. U.S.S.R. changing its constitution to democratic. (This country was disintegrated later on but remains a classic case as reason for disintegrating relates to the theory).
3. Struggle in European sub continent in non-democratic nations for change of leadership.
4. Nepal wanting to end the kingdom rule.
5. Urge for unification of Germany.
6. US using television gimmick to telecast their programme to the Cuban against the wish of their leader Freidel Castro.

7. Global consciousness for the depleting ozone layers and to reduce the emission of gases causing it.
8. Consciousness for preserving the nature and conserving the wild life.
9. Surgery of the unborn in the womb.
10. In the (Football) world cup history Cameroon team causing the upset in qualifying rounds of the match.
11. Gulf war-1 (which was in the process).

These are 15 years old story and so has become a part of history. All the above news items have the significance either with the mental evolution of the mankind or the steps taken up by the people of their country for the forward move or has significance with the logic sense where the scientist are always busy to meet tomorrows' demand. Many of the incidents have changed the scenario but the story continues.

Mental theory and the nations.

Let us see how we can put the nations in the mental theory and classify their state and analyse the right and the wrong steps being tried.

The mental frame for the (stable) national format is M-4. Today the entire world is distributed in different national set up. Nations are very small in territory, very big in territory; nations are with very high civilised state and very low civilised state of progress and so on. But by the mental theory all the nations have still not reached the M-4 stage and thus in this definition they are still not the nation.

What does this mean?

If they feel like nations they have to follow certain rule applicable in M-4 and if not the stability would be achieved only when they follow the rule applicable for M-3 or the mental frame they belong. There could be case where instability in a nation is observed but it could be a natural method to cross the threshold limit for the change over to reach the next mental frame for stability.

M-2: (Tribal format): Non of the countries would be in this category though there are lots of place within the countries existing today.

M-3: (Colonial format): We call present time as post - colonial era only because British or certain western rulers were ruling some part of the world and they have left that country. Leaving the country does not make it independent nation or at-least does not guarantee the mental rise, which is essential.

Most of the countries in Africa subcontinent and the gulf region would be in this category.

On the other side a small country with ample of money power and intelligence would also not qualify for M-3 status. Qualifying for this status would require more ingredients which they would lack because of less versatility available in themselves. Lots of European nations, which are quite small geographically tough rich and civilised would qualify for M-3 status. Though being in the higher civilised segment such nations would be having the urge to go up in the ladder (in their movement for contentment) but politically what step is required and how it has to be taken is of importance which restricts them in the lower mental frame.

Accordingly in M-3 mental frame distinctly we see one segment of nations with lower logic sense and the other segment with much higher logic sense. Are any of them satisfied? Both the segments would appear to have a stable system to the outside world but is it so?

M-4: United States is one true country to be classified. Indian subcontinent put together India and China also qualify with a slight variance.

M-5: No nation is in this category and no single nation would come. M-5 represents the culture and for that reason the world in the globalisation time of economy is also making the inclination to divide itself in distinct three cultures we read in the chapter-1.

U.S contributing for one culture is on the foremost runner in the race. For that reason India and China are said to be in M-4 level in variance which together could contribute to form a culture.

United States

United States is a country with people of the origin from different parts of the world. It is very big geographically. May be the people with higher mental frame chose come and settle here for what ever the reason. They are the foremost runner in the evolution of mental frame of the world. It means that they were the initial people to land in M-4 level mental frame and form a stable society known as a nation. They possessed all the ingredients required which have been mentioned for the positive process. As defined earlier it is the democratic behaviour of a nation which can lead to the openness and the positive path forward. But democracy needs further clarification because if it was so simple why did not other nations adopt.

Democracy does not mean easy going and all good things coming on their way. Such system has the greatest resistance to bring and adopt the changes in all the departments of civilisation within the country. US is said to be the biggest democratic run country because it has been able to give education to an average person to elevate their own mental frame. Higher mental frame means superior to others and having more logics to understand other human being and their need. On the other hand being in superior level also could lead the generation of superiority complex surfacing out the superficial ego in the individual level. The ego in the society of comparatively people of higher mental frame could lead to the clashes within them or outside the country.

US being the largest democracy has given the liberty to its people to work in the scientific areas for innovations in all the fields below the deep down sea to the living being on the earth, to the endless stars and galaxies. It is the democratic power, which has given the opportunity to attract people from the entire world to put their skills and contribute their effort in the scientific innovation. These people from around the world do not belong to different nations but belong to one breed of realised persons who require a basic platform to operate their mind and their talent. Their results and success stories are never any nation specific but are for the mankind. For this reason the scientists have explored all the avenues relating to the nature, body and the other world. The openness of the national system has allowed attracting people for development or acquiring the ideas innovated elsewhere for its utilisation for the larger mankind. It also gives the chance for a leader to be satisfied to see his countrymen first utilising the benefit. In such a set up of higher mental frame newer problems emerging out are taken as newer challenges and scientist and engineers are prepared for the solution. For example if the transportation is slower, faster and fuel efficient system is invented. If they come with newer disease or any physical complications they come up with new medicine or surgeries.

Though the progressing in the democratic way was a positive step the initial objective (few generations back) must have been very clear and well defined. With the concentrated development on the scientific area then the speed of the development was faster than demanded by the mass and till then it was not of concern. Further as there is always a difference of approach between the scientist and the general user. In this case many developed products which were made for the dedicators of the society to facilitate in their duties towards the mankind were seen as the product by the general user providing more physical and or mental comfort. With time and generation when these people of higher mental frame adopted these modes for their comfort probably they forgot what the suffering was. The process gradually made them so weak that they were not ready even to think how and why one suffers. The rat race started to necessarily have those comforts and their objective changed to acquire them. Next step was the fear looming around to live without these comfort modes made them run to do what ever needed towards it.

The democratic pattern of the country attracted the best technical brains form the world. The development was fast and the benefit was localised to a great extent rather than to be distributed in the larger mass. The obvious reason is to fulfil the national pride and giving the countrymen the pride of the best facilities available and invented. This was the transition period when the people with variance in degree of higher mental frame had the ability to *see* and *think* beyond and invent the need for time to come. The added facility could be useful necessary tool only to the dedicators for the society but there was no method to segregate such people. The newer facilities were available at cost and reduced the physical and mental load of the human. The situation changed the objective of an average human of this country to acquire the comfort. It did lead them to become more mobile and put extra hours in a day. The affect on people who were in not the appropriate mental frame for utilisation of all these was that it made them cross the threshold limit of life.

The threshold limit of the life is a state where one does not find a time to THINK at the real issues because one does not uses the required physical energy for the balancing of the act in self but over utilises the mental energy which would be negative to oneself. Crossing the threshold limit for mental rest the easiest way appear is the physical pleasure (which basically is an indication to him that extra physical energy in positive work would give satisfaction). Instead one mistakes for physical comfort.

The result of crossing the threshold speed of life has been that either people exploited physical charm for the comfort or on the other hand people with physical comfort felt relaxed with physical charm.

Let us focus on cause and effect in smaller units of individuals, families and organisations existing at higher mental frame that would have the impact in the country.

The elevated mental frame at the individual level stands for more of mental work and lesser physical work for the satisfaction. This situation itself calls for the reduction of population. This elevated mental place also requires the variation in the basic need of food habits. The food habits should be more refined to give less of labour to the body to work on it. Here there is a problem. If this fact is not understood and refinement is not brought a person would require more exercise to keep physically and mentally fit and would cause the delay in rising as the work may not be demanding enough physical exertion required. In the process in the readjustment period of body and mind in the new changed system would have the tendency to generate newer types of disorders and diseases beyond his knowledge.

This has caused the deviation of objective for the search of contentment and cannot sustain long enough. There are plenty of people who have started feeling the pinch and many have started the method towards the objective but with each time lapsed the equation keeps becoming complex. Once the threshold speed of life is crossed the contentment becomes very difficult. It can be gauged from the fact the what a 40 or 50 year old human desired today it is desired by a person of half the age and it does not stop there. With passage of time much younger and younger person wants to achieve what their peers tried much later in their life. Be it material or comfort or recognition every coming generation wants to do much sooner and thus they over rule the basic social norm set to keep the system in harmony.

The best part with the people of this land is that they were the first to step in the new path and were the first to experience it and thus it has the relevance to the entire mankind of the remaining world. Majority of the people would belong to higher mental frame with variance in degree and at this higher mental frame the real satisfaction could be achieved only by mental pleasure rather than the physical pleasure. Here the threshold speed of the life is a hurdle as well as a challenge for them to overcome it. If the human of this land have become independent of each other in the process they have become dependent of material. If the material need has made their economy sound it has made them realise that the natural resources have the limit and they would be the worst sufferers without them.

What could be the remedy?

This makes people think to either

i. Reduce the threshold speed of life where their acquired logic sense in the process and the ego of superiority remains as a hurdle or

ii. Go further up in the mental frame which is a realised state where the material and wealth for one does not mean more than to run his physical body and mind machine.

At the individual level many have started to find the ways. The different ways would vary from one own mental frame. Few examples are such as people joining social organisation for their service for poor irrespective of country, dedicating their life for wild life preservation. Spiritualization and meditation like teaching are there which could provide the ray of hope for contentment on the individual level.

By our elemental theory they were placed first in the outermost orbit where moral values were the key values required. But as a nation if we see the situation in U.S and with the process of the advancement and speeding of life they have formed a different culture of their own. Further going by our elemental theory it can be said that they have reached the situation where the moral values alone is no more sufficient for achieving the contentment. Moral values have started showing a drift that may appear to be ridiculous statement but is not in the context of elemental theory.

If we consider only the positive side of the elemental theory it is like fruit having multiple layer of values. First layer was pealed to find the love value. All other higher values had no importance for them. As they moved forward in their journey and were able to remove the second layer they encountered respect as the value. Here it becomes important to understand that if any individual or a unit is abiding a respect value (in its true meaning) the love value itself is contained and does not require separately to have this value. The love value does not become redundant but its isolated importance does become unimportant.

This would make understand that to cross the outer core level where moral values is situated the US needs to cross over and have to try to peal another layer of the fruit. It should be also understood that each forward keeps becoming more and more complex and so this time complexity is of highest order that mankind has come across. It should also be understood by a reader by now that when there is an urge to cross over there are distinct two paths positive and negative working simultaneously. If US has reached first till the outer core would they continue to lead? Could be or could be not. Time would tell that but what is happening can be explained as following.

From the national level they are situated in a higher mental frame and the present situation calls for having a sharp sense of humanity, which may be visible in certain sections of this society. There is equally or larger a negative force acting in the system. In either case moving positive or negative the importance of moral value is bound to reduce. The difference that in one case being at a higher new value it would be imbedded while in the other case it would show the loss. The question of moral values with reference to a nation has a sense when units other human network are dependent on each other in some way. But if units from biggest to the smallest become independent and even if they continue to work smoothly the moral value does not find the place and the smooth running system could be only a stopgap system. The affect of the culture is very much visible in the smallest unit that is a family. A man and woman who marry to call themselves husband and wife are equally independent need not have moral values for immediate survival. The self-independent has the flaw and does have the boon as well. The present situation of independence of every individual of people with varied mental frame is misnomer. Some may classify the culture having a different set of values but the reason is simple that in urge of every one finding a self-identity the have become dependent on material losing the sense of constitution which could do more harm. As described in the elemental theory shift of moral values or the constitution in the outer core where US is situated would cause them towards the physical changes. On the negative side it would mean physical attraction, physical satisfaction, physical relation and so on. Most of these people basically are of higher mental frame with embedded instinct of humanity so it becomes critical for them to make the shift towards the positive end and could be by associating with human being of the world beyond their country. There are people who are aware of this and see the defect in the system, such people are working for the larger community of the world for their own contentment and few of them could do wonders.

What about the average people?

Dependent or independent all are man made social set up. The loss of constitution has the affect in the lower units directly. As survival is natural instinct of every unit and in the national set up the lower unit has its role to play also. These units are social unit, farming sector, organisations which we have explained earlier. These units run on the respect as a core value. Now when the importance of constitution starts reducing these next lower units start showing a stronger respect value for mere survival. The respect which would appear to be growing stronger for survival becomes demanding and is in the conflict with the values when developed which were in commanding nature.

The demanding nature of the respect in turns start becoming physical. What is the outcome? The organisation turns professional. Here professional word has to be interpreted properly where in each social sector has a clear demarked area of work. His duty and earning is cared to fulfil the basic need and there is a dedication within an organisation with reference to the money earn for his living. Working on a specific format and defined duties could have fewer chances of improvement and could thus devoid the ability of self-development.

As professionalism defined is form of physical respect it cannot be the path for harmony, which is in the level of organisation (inner core of humanity) it has the effect down below in the smaller unit as well. The family is the unit where love is the core value and in turn we have observed that love also has turned physical. The need of material in this physical requirement has led to polluting the environment in more than one ways and average human only oversees it for his part of material gain.

The US is a place with the best brains. To find the solution of environment pollution is the problem of scientists who are a dedicated lot. As scientists are people working on logics they would search an alternative to nullify the ill effect by the way of improved technology or the change of a component or by sophistication in technology. But any option would be a mere physical art that a human can do at the best. The effect of sophistication and modified technique may give am immediate relief but would likely create a problem of higher magnitude, which would be realised after a long time gap.

Summarising the situation of US it has generated a western culture. The mental frame of the nation has gone above M-4. Mental level has gone at the level where even the moral values are not enough for the derivation of contentment unless a strong humanity instinct emerges in the nation. Superiority ego and dependence on material could be a roadblock but still they remain at the best level to work for the world unconditionally for their own survival.

How it could happen?

Tapping the humanity has the implication on all individuals, social or nations. As for the individuals they are supposed to be above the basic need and if they start looking after the share of love which is missing they could find it by feeding (providing the primary basic need) to the people who may be even outside their territory or even outside the nation. The assistance to a needy and a shear selfless attitude could only provide them the mental peace.

At organisational level the speed needs to be reduced. One way could be that instead of all individuals possessing surplus and organisation generating lots of profit one need to put a limit such that certain surplus produced could be shared with people outside their territory or the nation. The sharing with other nation may not be done free of cost but could be done similar to the barter deal. The material or cost in return to the deal could be decided by them as they are in the better and higher mental frame to suggest for any specific situation keeping their state in the mind. Such method not only would raise the mental level of those at the lower level but in the process could provide some spectacular ideas in business or the process which would make them grow more.

At the national level US is the most advanced democratic country and in the highest mental frame. Their mental frame M-4 is located where constitution (or moral value) is losing its importance and thus would be lacking the basic sense to generate the national spirit. But the mental level and scientific strength has a tendency to use its superiority to safe guard the world as their brothers and sisters and enlarge working beyond the national territory to win the hearts of the people of the world with different mental frame, different physical strength and different scientific strength. The process can fulfil their ego and generate the feeling lost.

Interpretation of the some news item related to US under 'testing the hypothesis' (mentioned in page 76 with addition of the latest news item)

(1) US using television gimmick to telecast their programme to the Cuban against the wish of their leader Freidel Castro. (Year 1989) We have said that the television is the most effective media for communicating the message to the masses. It works on a single-track method where miscommunication could lead in more than one way. US being on the higher mental frame can understand the difficulty of

people of undemocratic nation and could assume their plight by a dictating leadership. The nation can have the humanity feeling to help the people of such a place on the other hand but in this higher mental frame level people can not be satisfied by winning an opponent unarmed. Only because they have the resources and facilities of satellite and use its influence on the people against their own leader would be a negative utilisation of scientific idea that can only mis fire. The proper way could be only be if the message of democracy is passed through their leader and helping them to resolve the prevalent issues.

(2) Global consciousness for the depleting ozone layers and to reduce the emission of gases causing it. (1989) The news is old but is sill fresh. It does not only relate to US but to the entire developed world. One example such as chloroflurocarbons (CFCs) is assumed to be causing the effect of depleting ozone layer. One use of fluorocarbon (Freon) is in refrigeration, which for mass application. The scientist in the highest mental frame state have found the substitute and the fridges have started using the substitute gases. But what is the implication?

i. Would the substitute not harm the atmosphere? Scientifically one would be able to comment on it but if not directly it would have the implication after a time gap and the implication could be more sever.

ii. On the other side the substitute has to be costly and bearable by the people of nation above basic need and the one who are responsible for degrading the environment. There is another world, nations of lower mental frame which are in the state of increasing mental frame, for them even the domestic fridge was not a necessity but should become with time to come. The new costly fridge could further delay in the reach of a common man to save the world environment where as their contribution in damaging the environment is minimum. Some one is doing the ill and someone else is suffering for everyone welfare. Is it justified?

(3) Consciousness for preserving the nature and the reducing wild life. The US has the largest human in the higher mental frame. There they have the people above the basic need. There they have to concern about the world (at the individual level) and thus brought the conciseness about the reducing wild life and its preservation. The dedicated people are spending their lifetime even in the wildest jungle for the cause of the world tomorrow. In the process such people also help in raising the mental frame of the people lying much lower due to their natural placement in that world.

(4) Surgery of the unborn in the womb. (News 1989) The US being in the highest mental frame have dedicated scientist we have already explained. The scientists are working with the vision of tomorrows need. Therefore most of such medical inventions are to happen there. Scientist could belong to any country but the national freedom for any achiever to give the opportunity is large. Such scientist feet would be for any human but the requirement would be only to the people situated in higher mental frame because of losing their certain natural strength.

(5) Gulf war-1 (1989 which was in the process when the essay was written initially). The Gulf war-1 was on the 26th day of its progress. In our concept the US is above M-4 where as Kuwait and Iraq would fall maximum in M-3 category. The war by US shows the intent to help Kuwait against Iraq for its sovereignty, which is a part of the humanity at the national level. The step taken though is a negative one. If the initial purpose was to scare Iraq by virtue of being in the level mental frame emphasising her superiority physically which is not making an ego issue with Iraq. At the existing mental

frame US cannot be first to start the war, as they would have more fear for people getting killed or hurt even if they out win the war. If the war is anyway started first the decision could have taken in absence of balanced thought in subconscious and for the act US might have to repent for much time to come ahead.

In the war face to face physically they cannot win as they are inferior in physical strength but with sophisticated technology and instruments and from a very far distance they can be devastating also. Their target could be more on humanity ground involving more on material and less on humans. On the other hand Iraq is in different mental frame where people have more physical strength and would have more dedication spirit for their leader. If such people get latest weapons even if they are not sophisticated as their opponents can harm more and have the ability to win the territory. They cannot be blamed for having ego instead if they were given proper respect and heard about their problem the issue could have materialised more easily.

Where is the situation going to lead?

The question is not who wins and who was correct as in a fight any party cannot be said to be correct and any justification cannot convince them morally for the act. If the negative step has been taken place and the stability has been disturbed the case becomes interesting. By our theory Iraq is at M-3 and they have to stay thee or go up for the search of contentment. In next 20 days or next 20 years the real stability lies only when they move towards M-4 level. To reach at such position Iraq may not remain Iraq or Kuwait as Kuwait but there may be a cultural amalgamation to give a national set up and reach the level of M-4. Where as US lies at or above M-4 where contentment lies in humanity it is realise by them. If physically lose the war their superiority ego becomes predominant and once the negative tactic of war has started it is not possible that they see it as lost battle. If some how peace is brought it would be a temporary phase but the subconscious has to come out to win at that place or even somewhere else. This winning game felt by some part of the world could only lead to barbaric inhuman tactics, which could create more of devastation. The devastation caused could lead to realise the loss of humanity and thus help to elevate in the mental frame in search of the contentment. The humanity would mean to have the moral values and respect with other nations and see their basic needs are met.

(6) Gulf war-I1 (August 2004). As written above the peace would be only a temporary phase the gulf war happened once again. Their leader Saddam Hussain is captured and more important the nation is injured badly. Which country has achieved what is not clear but both US and Iraq have disturbed the existing peace and possibility ahead is,

US: Even if they feel the pain and try to be more human the negative step taken has made their path for contentment of a nation complicated and it would not be able to achieve without the support of some other segment of the world, which is placed in similar mental frame without inflicting such wounds in herself. In the due course US will have to shelve the superiority ego and use its mental and scientific resources for the other world. As a rule for going up in the humanity level US should spread the culture with positivity beyond the national level and the larger cultural segment works for the betterment of the needy section of our world. Probably at present it has lost the opportunity to do by itself.

Iraq on the other hand, which was lying at or below M-3 mental level with its disturbed peace, has an opportunity to go up in the ladder. This cannot happen by itself. There are many nations around Iraq in the similar mental frame. The route to the stability could come when few of these nations combine with different culture together when that group as one can truly come in the national format and rise towards mental M-4 for the stability. But if rule is not followed and instead small countries combining to give the national format and if that region tries to find the peace by joining in a cultural format it would be not correct. There is no short cut and they have to step in M-4 level and the cultural level for humanity is allocated for M-5. They forming a cultural segment at this stage could only be negative for themselves.

European Countries

US find itself in a specific higher place as nation in values and logic sense because of various factors it possess we have discussed. The nation is able to make a culture out of it. We call it western culture and culture itself means that it has the tendency to spread beyond the national boundaries. Where do the European countries stand in the context?

Europe consists of many nations and almost all of them (baring Russia) are quite small in the territory. Mostly country have fewer religion mix of people to have the affect in the national system. Mostly are in good economical condition and most would be having the ruling system appearing nearer to the democratic function.

We would define in general term rather than individually and for that points related of concern are

- Nations in absence of multi-language and multi religion misses some vital part of experience of tolerance, sacrifice and patience in the national level.
- Even the democratic behaviour in smaller nation end up in a kingdom sort of rule as it does not give enough variables to tackle of a larger nation.
- Few nations not confirming to democratic rule had to change themselves.

The European nations along with many other nations in

American and south Asian continent with similarity are in a complex state. In these nations individuals or the lower social units (organisations and the family) have reached M-4 mental frame where as the nation itself is lagging and could be said in or above M-3 level. The culture acquired is like western and concerns to them from the national point of view. If at individual have reached M-3 level the contentment route is humanity and for that reason making or amalgamating to a culture beyond the national boundary is understandable but what about the nation which is lagging as a unit? It cannot bring the harmony and thus we call it a complex state.

Simultaneously if many nations in this land are observed as a one unit it still does make a better sense. The nations being at a lower level would have fear of security of any kind even if they have good neighbours. The insecure national status could inculcate the insecurity in the individuals also though not necessarily. Let us observe some different political decision relating to it.

(1) Common Euro currency: As these nations are at or above M-3 level and have better economic conditions one way to lift them to M-4 is by making one unit in the trading with outside world. It could make them feel more secure. This cohesion on trade relate to the higher logic sense and its application towards the goal but would it answer the human inter relation within them is still a question.

(2) UK supporting US. UK is a part of Europe and a nation, which had occupied a major part of the world once. It brings them in the superiority ego and so feel good factor with the superior nation on the day only fulfils a false sense of security. It could do more effective role with other European nations.

(3) France: Is the nation where the people are bold to talk about what they perceive without the fear. In the

context of gulf war-II France was first to speak against UK and US for starting the war unilaterally. Many other European nations must have felt same but did not confront for their own selfish gain. Such statement by a nation relating to global issues without the fear calls for the urge of humanity and could be one contender to lead this group and find a method to make the nations reach M-4. There are infinite examples to prove where within the western culture France has been vocal and negative on many issues. Their guts to talk in negative about the global issues calls for the leadership within the segment and thus would guide Europe to the unknown path but would leave on other nation to complete the task.

(4) Germany: One of the other nations could be Germany.

The negative path for the contentment appearing to be shorter by an individuals or any unit could be only an illusion ad in fact would become a longer one. He positive path, which may appear to be very tedious and complicated, is shorter and the one, which could be the one to keep the civilisation, survive.

West Germany with its people at higher mental frame than the national mental frame has set an exemplary case for up-liftment towards the nation and also the humanity which should be opener for US also. W Germany is a democratic nation with western culture and higher logic sense. History would reveal that this part of the world had one of the richest civilisation (place of Aryans) and in logic sense it were the German people most advanced which US and Russia has stolen for their advancement. This background of a nation could only take a small step which was value based. The nation understood their problem in search for the contentment and where individual units situated at higher mental frame could have opted for the path of spiritualization but that could not have lead to the growth and basic existence of the civilisation. Instead they have opted to slow down the speed of life by unification with East Germany.

The effect of unification in values

Unification means sacrificing their extra share for the people or their brothers and sisters. East Germany on one hand was not a democratic governed nation and thus there was a lag in the mental frame of the nation and their people meeting with people who are experiencing the self-independence at the individual level having higher speed of life. In such a situation East Germany finding the new freedom could tend to increase the speed of life without even coming in the state of self independent could have a snag. This could tend to break the moral values at the national level before as a nation comes in M-4 level by the people falling in the physical and material lust, which West Germany has realised as no-good and crossed over. If West Germany would find contentment in sacrificing for their brothers and sisters- the lost love – mistaken respect - and misunderstood constitution would start falling in its place.

On the other hand if East Germany would be attracted for the physical values, close contact with their counter part would make them realise the role of the life very soon. In the process they could try to acknowledge it with more neighbouring countries around and could benefit in improving the national mental frame and proceed for humanity ahead. This is one possibility of positive way to move ahead and at least could unify the Europe as one culture.

The effect of unification in logic sense

German were with the greatest human minds in technology and thus they have equally to worry on the global issues such as

- increasing ozone layer,

- depleting nature and wild life,
- surgery of unborn in the womb etc.

We have read that in the process of becoming independent people have become dependent of material (which we have termed as western culture) as the speed of their life has increased. Once human is accustomed to man made things rather than human himself newer medical problems keep cropping. It means in the process of utilising the natural resources because of his dependence on it he becomes weaker physically. Now united Germany has opted the path, which would slow down the threshold limit of the speed. As they have the interest in realising the sacrifice it is the process where they would have the inclination to become dependent on their brothers and sisters. Unlike US their mental frame for spiritualization would be not directly towards God but towards the God's creation with other humans followed by other living being's and the nature.

This is the mental frame where their regular movements would be like one learns in yoga. Inclination towards yoga, learning and spreading of yoga would be done by masses. Such activities would eat away the time which a mind otherwise would have wasted in the physical lust making them more positive. The people would be generally in good health but still would fall sick and would have physical problems. In the scientific advanced age the medicines and the surgeries are being developed and improved daily. It is the sharp logic sense which allows them to penetrate through the intricacies and come out with the results. Appreciating the achievements is one thing that may allow some to live for many more years. They would go further deep to trace the root cause for the problems and question,

- why every other day a new medicine is required or
- why situation should arise for example for a surgery of unborn in a mother's womb.

The scientific achievement and the doctors expertise can be strength for the suffering patient but the question of why is generated because of the fat man may go wrong man made things may go wrong but the nature cannot go wrong. For this reason if something in the natural process is going wrong it is only man himself to be blamed and thus the answer is the quest and to be found.

An average person in this world is going upward in the mental frame in his or her own reference. As one goes up even slightly his physical potential is reduced and becomes physically weaker and with half or improper knowledge about his ailment makes him mentally weaker also. For example a patient is detected suffering with a cancer which is detected in a very early stage of its growth. Here if one comes to know about deadly cancer the knowledge might create a fear and make him mentally so week that he would never recover where as if a patient does not know in medical term and develops a higher mental frame he would overcome and the disease would vanish. West Germany as a nation is in such a mental frame which could work wonders for human values in science also. For this reason the Germans would more tend to accept the aurvedic medicines over the conventional allopathic as the root medicine. Thus slowing the threshold speed of life and moving ahead in their mental frame would bring up the technology of aurvedic and could show the world a positive way.

One of the news item mentioned:

In the (Football) world cup history Cameroon team causing the upset in qualifying rounds of the match. (News 1989)

Cameroon was in the lower mental frame comparing to some other countries in the fray. In the process of rising in the mental frame one loses its physical strength to some extent.

This is to say if two person equal in all other respect are face to face except different mental frame the one in lower would win in any physical activity where as the other would win in the mental activity. In such a situation people belonging to higher mental frame are likely to loose the game with time. It should be known that for person selected be of higher mental frame is of lower mental frame at the individual level but if all of the nation go up they have to lose in the physical part be it the games.

Cameroon upsetting the European giants could not be considered as unusual. Football being a game requiring physically fitness and stamina if physically stronger people add the talent definitely they can upset other countries.

With this reference we can see how the rules in the sports have been twisted time after time to suit higher mental frame because of their superiority feeling.

Take an example of cricket: In the early days England and Australian how played the most are known for bowling bouncers which could cause injury and even death to a player. All such tactics were valid till few countries ruled and continue to retain their superiority. More countries participating would have given those leading countries a sense of higher superiority if they continue to be on the top. The emerging countries who happened to be on the lower mental frame and thus having more physical strength could have injured more people of the leading countries and reduce their ego. But the rules have been changed to reduce the bouncer, reduce to height of bouncer and so on and further framing the codes for penalising the player also. Changing the rules for the better is ok but sportsman spirit prevailed in the game till few countries were bending the rule for their convenience and when others joined the definition of sportsman ship changed.

The amendment of rules we can continue to observe to suit nations of higher mental frame in any international sports.

Countries switching for a Democratic set up

Let us take example of two countries distinctively apart politically.

1. USSR
2. Nepal

1. USSR. Today it is no more a USSR but fragmented into different pieces and RUSSIA being the biggest of them. The word USSR is written, as it was still not fragmented when this essay was originally written in 1989. The description detail of a USSR on the basis of mental frame, which was conceived by the author 15 years ago and is written as then below in italics,

USSR is a typically a complicated case. It has been one of the major super power but still not democratic till sometime back. The scientific development has allowed there to acquire more logic sense which was contributed to raise the mental frame for the few individuals but the national system being socialist has forced the them to live in groups with interdependency. This pattern makes a situation where at the individual level the mental frame would be in very wide spectrum (between M-1 to M-5) but the mental frame of the nation is far below (near or below M-3). The rise of logic sense would lead to finding the self-independence as a lasting end (which we have observed in the case of US and has resulted in generating a culture). The behaviour in USSR has been forcibly curbed and so the lasting end has not been achieved. What could likely happen at the individual level is that persons at higher mental frame would see the silver lining and could generate the independent feeling and would have high human values. The possession of humanity could be seen as a weak point and could be exploited by another lot at lower mental frame who see the new freedom as a tool to unload the stored and curbed ambitions by the easier path. The situation would lead to the changes in the molecular level and thus at the individual level there would be exploitation within the nation and at the national level the ego of being superpower would hamper.

The remarkable difference with the US can be gauged as following:

- *While in the case of US the nation has reached at higher mental frame, simultaneously the logic sense increase and the speed of the life has brought the situation where people can try to seek the contentment in working for other nations where as*
- *In the case of USSR the threshold speed has gone up with the logic sense but the national mental frame being at lower stage the contentment region is not beyond the national level.*

Result, the nation could be too dependent on other countries, which is just reverse to the state of US.

(After 15 years)

USSR has disintegrated into many pieces. We would call many nations but all such fractions would still not be able to meet the requirement for a national level from our theory. Russia is the biggest block, which would qualify for upgrading the mental frame at the national level. It has to shed the superiority ego and learn from Germany for that instant. At or above M-4 level nation generates a culture for moving ahead in the ladder. As Russia lagged in the mental frame they could only equate with the western culture rather than make one of their own. With the influence of western culture the urge of element for self-independence could be a wrong step which the aware people would realise. What the nation requires is the efficient utilisation of materials, which calls for generation of sacrifice and patience sort of elements within the people. Such values would be realised from the eastern culture existing around their geographical space but would be difficult to follow it. If till now they were not even in the M-4 level the nation will have to jump above the level in a short time (to match the logic sense) and again it would be the value of interdependency of human and social network would be realised as a media for contentment which till now had been forced on the people. It might take one or two generation to reach across mental frame M-4 but before that there would be lot of turbulence in the path. In such a complex situation the president of Russia or even last president of USSR could be one of the world's most realised leader to understand the co relation between the scientific development and the human values of a nation and its people and could have the remedy for the entire world. He might have a vision for a path of global peace and the vision towards the contentment for all the segments of the world but ironically he may not find the time to look beyond the country and exploit his vision for global harmony in his lifetime.

The other smaller nations of broken USSR remain or elongate the time to raise their mental frame and so are not important in our study.

2. Nepal:

Nepal is nation in the Himalayan region and between India and Tibet. Nepal could be insignificant to influence the world in any area but its urge to go democratic in their small world is a good example for our case study. Nepal, which we call as a nation in the today's history is barely near in M-3 mental frame or below for its kingdom type governance and even for its geographical small area. This nation lags in the logic sense also. In the state of colonisation it is the respect value the route for achieving contentment but the surrounding influence of the countries, which are far ahead, cannot give the peace. The nation comes across peoples' movement for a change against the ruler. The change could be a simple thought of some to bring them in democratic governance in a positive direction. Some could think to break the nation but such a step in such a small nation is not going the help any body.

For the former assumption to be true the nation has to rise in logic sense or could be possible by becoming a part of adjoining nations thus losing its own identity. The later assumption does not hold true for an additional reason. The nation irrespective of their mental frame has a strong influence by the eastern culture in and around the region. The eastern culture has the difference from the western culture from interdependency of one another in different smaller and bigger social units irrespective of rising in higher mental frame. Nepal has to come in stale M-3 mental frame and then move upwards to compete with others lying on the higher mental frame. There is only way for Nepal to rise keeping its identity is to keep the cultural association with neighbours which allows to enrich individual towards spiritual platform where any person with any degree of basic need and security can attempt to seek it to find a sense of contentment. With such force existing in the individuals they could have feeling as apart of the adjacent countries without the drive of self-independency.

India

We have said that U.S is in M-4 state contributes for generating one set of culture in the world and is the foremost runner in the race. We have also said that India and China are again in M-4 level in variance, which together could contribute to form another set of culture in the world. Let us understand India and its position.

India is the second biggest democratic nation in the world. If US has given western culture India is one of the biggest contributory in the development of eastern culture, which could be a guiding factor for other existing cultures for seeking the contentment. India is a nation with quite a big territory to be said as a nation. Bigger territory leads to have different mixes of human being and if they can live in unity in diversity there has to be a guiding force. India is one of the most populated nations in the world. India has poorest of poor and richest of rich people. There are many languages and many more sub languages spoken. The nation has many religions and many sub-religions. All put together it makes a homogeneous mixture of human network of all the evolution era with all degree of logic sense prevailing in sections and thus people of different mental frame. This makes a nation complex but simultaneously there hidden values binding all the segments. On the nature front there is extreme whether of hot and cold in summer and winter. There is plenty of rain in some parts where as droughts are there year after year in certain region. In such natural variance catastrophes have taken the lives and acted as boon for other to overcome it. The nation has forest and jungles on one end where as desert is also there. The natural mix is also responsible for the variance in the growth of mental frame of people within the nation.

There are pockets where tribes still exist; there are sections where values are at the tribal level and there is a large interphase in between where people know that love is the most significant binding force. Even if they are termed backward and uneducated they have enormous physical ability and if they do entirely physical job in their daily rituals they are satisfied in their engagements. Their mental frame does not have significance with reference to a nation and it does not matter to them which country they belong. The logic sense rise has been very low and thus speed of their life is very slow. In the context of today's advancement age they may belong to very deprived and inferior cadre and may appearing contributing hardly any thing in the development of society and thus the nation. Nevertheless the advance people of the same nation have something to learn from them and it is the love bond imbedded within them to keep survival in the artificial life and unnatural environment created by the other advanced section. If someone learns the positive values, which they still possess certainly, that section would impart the knowledge, which the tribal people lack and would lead to the contentment to both of the section.

In the social segment where organisation is also a part India has plenty of self-entrepreneurs in different mental frame and of different types. At the lower segment there are skilled craftsman who have talent, who work hard and generate novel material. This segment achieved the contentment in the hard work even when they do not get return from the labour they do. They have been at the exploited end by the broker (selling agents) who have been making the fat profits they have been exploited by the modern machinery stealing there business but still have been transmitting the art from one generation to the other. Such people have probably reached higher mental frame but the logic sense remains lower to be satisfied. There is another segment of entrepreneur with small-scale industries put up by comparatively higher mental frame people. They belong to the area where love (or basic need) could cause harmony between few employee and the employer and thus raise the mental frame of the unit by producing quality product and generating more profits to grow further. The entrepreneurs who are able to define the basic need and the functional duties of the working force and able to bring a proper equilibrium are the one who are able to sustain the growth and reach to the stage of organisation where few working force increases such that the respect value becomes more important in the inter human relation. They are also the people who rise in the mental frame and show the path to the others connected along with the rise of logic sense as much required to the individuals.

On the other side there are plenty of such people who work on short-term basis who do not care for the values. This lot has raised the logic sense much higher than required and thus create problem for themselves along with the people associated with them.

The farming sector is similar to the colonial era where the prime force is the respect. The social norms in this segment made had in depth significance for people and by people. This is most stable platform ever made which could keep the mankind survive with nature and could also take care of the values along. The speed of the life has been under the threshold limit and so the contentment has been in the visible range. The absence of inadequate infrastructure for elevating the mental frame by education has made a lot of gap between the people to cause the insatiability in the peaceful small world. For improving the mental frame some migrate towards the city for good and bad in absence of proper knowledge and some extend their leadership instinct in the same area. Both of these movements have different effect on the national level as a whole. There has been internal exploitation of the people and by the people.

Where as in the urban side the industrial boom has allowed to elevate the logic sense and consequently attack the nature. The industries, which operate on the strength of respect value similar to the colonial form have given varied experience. The industries which have cared for the values have not only risen economically but have been successful in satisfying the people in and out (employee, customer and all other associated) and developed a culture to upgrade their mental frame. There are industries not following the natural law have worked for short term gain which have cause disturbance in the culture attacking the nature without knowing the consequence and even closing down their organisation at time. Elevation of mental frame has taken place of all with generations of such movement. The movement has also allowed the people to give the knowledge of both positive and negative results making them to think for a process to find a platform where the speed can be limited below the threshold limit to keep them contended.

The beauty of the Indian democracy is that the freedom of thinking and acting in all the sections in the individual capacity. This has allowed the flourish the next group of people whose mental frame is higher at M-4 level who operate above the national system on the humanity level. Thus

i. Scientific achievers who were far from sufferings have shown wonders outside India.
ii. The segment that knew the sufferings has been propagating humanity not only within the nation but globally.
iii. One realise segments in this group without the attachment of name and fame have been working selflessly uplifting the society in all walks of the life.

There is another (advanced) sections generated logic sense and the speed of life has crossed the threshold limit and this lot is only getting confused, as they have to interact with their counterpart at the slower speed. This section tends their approach towards the western culture but the satisfaction could be achieved if a large part is influenced to isolate as western culture. Even if a small section in isolation feels the satisfaction it would realise only as a stopgap platform from where actual path for the contentment could be seen gone farther away. In the decade time the advanced section would realise that majority will not change their culture to the western and thus would cause the emergence of redefined culture which would remain eastern and would be the guiding factor to others.

Normally the mental frame of nation is around one level among M-2, M-3 or M-4 and minor sections above and below the existing one. This general situation has a sense for its existence, which indicates that either culture of a nation is one. The method reaching could be two (1) if the national mental frame falls on the higher side by the uniform growth and democratic methods and (2) by the mental frame falling on the lower side if the leadership instincts have been curbed by the non democratic functioning of a nation.

These two cases infer that the nation is governed either by the mental force of the people (as in the former case) or by the physical force of the people (as in the later case). The situation of India is very different where all the mental frames exist in sufficient quantum and still is able to generate one culture. It can be said the physical force is being acted in a part where the mental force in another. Overall the nation still as one unit only implies that it is the people who are governing the nation and not the other way round.

Even if we see historically Portuguese have invaded, Muslims have ruled and British have governed. All of them have gone but have left their impression and none could break the nation. There must have been some internal force to sustain and stay alive as a nation.

How do all the mental frame exist and maintain a culture?

This can be viewed from two perspectives which separates second biggest Indian democracy from US which is the biggest democracy of the world,

1. US was able to lift mental frame of large section of its people by making them feel above the basic need and thus improving the logic sense of the nation. The result was that stronger economic nation exploited the other section of the weaker world. Where as in India the exploitation has been within the nation by one section of the people to another section of the weaker section. In the former case the realisation in the individuals may not creep where as in the later case with generation realisation could appear in either section being together.

2. The nation has been soaked with Hindu religion so deeply that even different mental frame people found satisfaction in their route for achieving contentment. The rise of logic sense did not come in priority and slow speed of life did not deter their way of life.

We understand that the ultimate goal of any individual or colony or nation at any mental frame is contentment. Breaking further in the individual level the contentment is the mental state easily obtained by the spiritualization. The spiritual bent in the lowest mental frame has allowed not to speed up their life as contentment appearing visible within their scope with lesser needs. We know that mental frame of individuals and the nations only rise and never come down. Thus segment whose mental frame rises with time are still able to realise the contentment in the path of spiritualization.

In case of India the rise at the individual level has been slower. Spiritualization has a place at all the mental frames and even at lower mental frames of M-2 and M-3 it has a tendency to know more about humanity. This character has generated clash within a mind of one section that are trying to follow western culture and not changing the existing culture. The slow speed of life and higher mental frame has generated a segment to write about the changing socials as a mean to communicate to the people, generated a segment creating live in art, music and dance and poetries which could keep open the eyes of people about the wrong steps they have taken as a chance to reform themselves.

The overall situation of India is that where exploitation of highest degree is happening within the nation on one end humanitarian work is also being carried. A big section in mental frame M-2 in such a set up could bring demanding leadership activities but that could be short lived and in the process generate a commanding leader as well. Such a leader could even influence the developed world for peaceful coexistence in this universe and he could shakes hand with China with whom they could be able to demark the culture globally to guide the rest of the world.

China

China is classic example for the study, which has so much to give to rest of the world for coexistence. It has been communist governed nation and lately have changed towards the democratic way. The democracy percolation would take lot of time to the average people. China is influenced with Buddhist culture, which has kept the people satisfied in spite of strict political regime so far.

The Hindu religion in India and Buddhist religion of China have the potential to transform the Eastern culture in this part of the world against the western culture existing in US, Europe and many other advanced nations. In this culture the human inter-dependency at various levels of family and other social pockets can not be ruled out over material. In this populated nation even if the logic sense has gone up which has a tendency to speed up the life the un-democratic nature of governance has been responsible to slow down the speed and maintain a harmony. As a nation only democratic framework can pave path in positive development and so China at last has tried to change the functioning. True the change or the fruit would not reach the lowest section immediately and so the process would take many generations to creep the benefit to all. The freedom at the individual level could lead to internal exploitation, some section could be influence by the western culture with bringing the openness in the system but the Buddhist religion would again restrain the people to shift and leave their own culture. Till now the strictness of the communist system has given the realisation of discipline at the individual level, which is one tool to derive contentment and has been missing in the case of India.

Discipline in the individual level maintains the harmony in the society and is like shock absorber to bear all the hardships to maintain the norms of human interdependency. In case of China it has not been the political system force to bring the discipline, which could have been broken long time back. It is the religious bent which has allowed following the norms which are responsible to bring the contentment in all the mental frames with their knowledge, skills and their need

The African Continent

This part of the world has peculiar state. African continent has nations which lag behind in the progress human has made and also in mental frame. The remotest areas still have typical tribal people to educate the developed world about their habitats. If the human progress has been slow they have fewer values to work with, they have a lesser demand of material and have been maintaining the environment balanced. Certain nations have the rich nature of forest with varieties of species of animals under the fear of extinction elsewhere which the advanced world admire. If South Africa has been explored by the advanced world for the natural wealth Egypt has a background of strong culture and so has been on the higher mental frame comparatively. These can be the most influential for the upliftment of remaining nations. Most of the nations apart can be said existing around the M-2 mental frame. If they are lagging in the advancement with the other world they have also to give certain values which advanced section tend to lose in the process of speeding the life. From the mental theory these nations are far from being called a nation by themselves and can not influence the world for a long time yet.

Gulf Nations

The developed people of the developed world who have become independent of other human being have become dependent on material. Petroleum oil is one most important thing which people are dependent. Gulf region is known to be having big reserves to dictate the developed world. Ironically the nations around here have been in the eyes of the developed people for the resource available. The nations still have the kingdom sort of rule and probably to have the hold on the oil it could have been easier to influence a king rather than a professional nation. The result is that developed countries try to keep the influence, the nations have generated wealth but still as a nation they have yet to grow. The area is under

Islamic religion, which has an old history for its glory. In such a state individuals who raise the logic sense and values would find their own country less to contribute for the national cause. On the other hand because these nations have generated wealth though in pockets and not growing in mental frame find in a similar situation as USSR as one nation at some time. Though individual nations have not reached M-3 mental state and so have not reached the pace where we can call them a nation in combined form are in conflict with themselves. They have the opportunity by combining all or many together to form one nation where all the values in a larger segment can come in picture and they can grow faster and in positive direction.

Few global issues of importance on the day

(1) 9/11 Twin tower crash: The conflict of ego between a superpower which has created a separate culture and a section with cultural confusion who want to impose their rule on others without going through the sequence of steps to improve the values and the logic and reach the same level to command rather than demand. A segment could be confused and could confuse many more is not important as the other party in conflict which is the biggest democracy in the world. The nation with biggest democracy in the world has to take care of the responsibility to lift others. Not fulfilling this could have selfishness and could bring the negativity in the approach and make many foes.

(2) Outsourcing: There is always something naturally would occur to guide the universe for a logical and unknown growth of human civilisation. In the context of the study of USA we said that the early democracy of the nation has brought major section of her people to live above the basic need of food and shelter. It is on the other end that people / community / have much more wealth than they can absorb or require. The solution to this is that extra is distributed to the needy which can be outside their country. Distribution by the country if the primary step it could have been called a very

noble step, which could have given them a commanding respect by the world. As a natural way of progress the situation has reached that the wealth is being distributed to the other part of the world, which is the demand of the time. Today outsourcing is affected in few advanced nations and similar things would affect other nations who would generate wealth more than their requirement and not share with the rest.

Conclusion

The laws of values applicable are identical in one unit, in two units or more than two units. The unit size could be of any size. The unit is the collective strength smallest being is one individual followed by a family. An organisation small or big, a nation or the world could be seen as one integral unit. But as the unit size keeps increasing within them additional values are required by breaking one unit into few sub units. No two human are identical and they view a same thing from two different angle and so two different set of larger units could view a same thing from a different perspective enlightening both (for making progress in their task) or creating a rift (slowing the progress without their knowledge). There ladder in logic sense which has led the scientific development requires to be matched with the value persisting for the unit for a balanced state. This is to say with the progress in values the logics should be increased which requires evaluation by the concerned unit for its well being. Higher value and lower logic sense or visa versa requires balancing act for every one well being.

The civilisation growth which we have described has been a human mental evolution and has grown in a systematic way similar as a tree. The growth pattern is thus a design of a much superior craftsman which would continue to happen. It was the human mind that was opened up right in the very beginning thousands of years ago which is still in the process of developing. It started with the basic knowledge, experimenting and applying the basics in different forms of values and logic sense and generating more knowledge which still continues to be done. The new mental zone has the unique inherent quality of duality which we have observed in the process of advancement facing two propositions of good or bad, positive or negative. Though the negative element as one branch nurtured with time has generated a strong leadership instinct but have lost some thing from the other branch opted the other direction. With each steps of progress the branches kept increasing except one that kept moving with the positive theme. We have come in age where the nation is a largest single body for worth comparison. Democracy is a positive way and many nations would be in the democratic way of functioning but one would be the real with unbroken chain to guide the rest not in the quest to conquer the world but to unify them.

The quest of the story was value v/s money power. The idea of the author was to find out that with the speed of the change of the world what would make win the race the money or the value?

At an individual level there is general understanding of the people that one who possess wealth is assumed to be happier. The understanding is also true that the people who followed certain values have only appeared to be victims of the system. Though money remains important as the food it is the value that has superseded but for a hard working individual or group or society or a nation the money would automatically come equivalent to the requirement of basic need. We have observed that with the growth of civilisation importance of individual and their glory does not have a part to play. It is the largest segment, which is critical as the nation in our present age. The irony is that by the mental frame theory there are few places, which can be designated as nations, which automatically would lead to their governance methodology gradually adopting democratic way directly or by experiencing the other way. As it would be understood that nation is only the intermediate step before the human, to bring every one of us in the same level in the same one world.

But the scientific development does not proceed so fast to create unknown worry of human devastation.

One last thing would not be as important on the day is that presently the evolving human mind is in the last lap of its peak.

What after that?

Crossing over the mind one would enter in the new world of intelligence. The realisation of mind would develop the understanding of intelligence which would be a new experience to the mankind. The intelligence spectrum would be again of area of duality but at a different and much higher platform.

What does this mean?

There would be a change in the logics as viewed from a intelligence platform compared to that as viewed from a mental platform. All the big adventures and inventions which we are proud of are of physical in nature as an end product would start appearing so natural and of much less importance. The evolution game would re-start similarly from a different base level. All that the human has achieved in a physical form would be then tried in a different form, much higher form. It starts with dreaming and are people have started dreaming towards that and are preparing to enter a new world.

The values would still remain the same which in any case requires to be enriched in the entire mass. It could be a big task, it could appear an impossible task and therefore we have to wait for a visionary of that calibre to emerge to show the path.